CARB CYCLE

BY FRANCO CARLOTTO

CONTENTS

CHAPTER FIVE:

CHAPTER SIX:

CHAPTER SEVEN:

CHAPTER EIGHT:

CHAPTER NINE:

CHAPTER TEN:

APPENDIX:

INTRODUCTION

WHO IS FRANCO CARLOTTO?

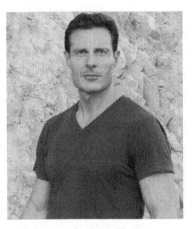

For those of you who don't know me, I have had the extreme fortune of earning the title of Mr. World Fitness not once or twice, but six consecutive times. Training for and winning the Mr. World Fitness competition was the culmination of a two-decade journey, and throughout the course of these last 27 years I have gained the knowledge enabling me to present you the truth about achieving optimal fitness.

Over the years, I've experimented with every possible diet and exercise routine ever invented. I've learned the hard way what really works and what doesn't. Because of this, I can give you the immediate benefits of my research and experimentation and you will never have to go on another frustrating diet or exercise program ever again. Whether you want to lose weight, maintain weight, get in great shape, are interested in training for athletic competition, or simply want to adopt a healthier lifestyle, my diet and exercise system will inspire you to make your dreams a reality and give you all the tools necessary to change your life. Most importantly, I will give you my revolutionary take on nutrition by introducing you to my Carb Cycle System, which is the most powerful diet ever developed for burning fat and getting in great shape.

I assure you, I have the experience to guide you in the right direction. Before I became Mr. World Fitness, I tried and studied low-fat diets, low-carb diets, no-carb diets, high-carb diets, different carb cycle techniques, high-protein diets - everything you can think of. **What I finally discovered in the 90's was a special way to eat and cycle certain carbs that literally forces your body to burn fat in an on-going, never-ending Cycle.** I called my secret: **CARB CYCLE.** Once I implemented this revolutionary approach to eating carbs, everything changed. Not only did I win the Mr. World Fitness contest, I won it six consecutive times. No one else could match my fitness level, because no one else had my eating secret. While my competitors wasted their time and money on complicated fitness programs and difficult diets, I got lean and in shape while still eating rice, bread, oatmeal, pasta, and potatoes with all my meals - exactly the stuff that most "experts" say you can't eat to get in great shape.

Now that I'm retired from competition, I've settled in Los Angeles, where I teach my (R)Evolutionary Carb Cycle Method to all kinds of people – celebrities, athletes, housewives, seniors - and let me tell you, everyone I share this secret diet with is getting amazing results! And now, for the first time ever, I want to share it with you and the world too. That's why I've written this book that I guarantee will make you understand fitness and dieting once and for all. It will enable you to lose weight and stay in shape like never before. Now, you may have looked at my pictures and be thinking, "I can never get my body even close to that kind of shape." Don't worry about that right now. Just know that what I will be revealing to you will not intimidate you. Instead, it will motivate you to be the best you can be. I guarantee you that you too can get your body into great shape based on your individual build and the revolutionary concept that I will teach you. Regardless of your current physical condition, I am confident that my Carb Cycle will help you get into your best shape ever, and teach you how to maintain it for life!

Once you read this book and learn how to re-arrange the exactly right carbs on this safe, logical, and most efficient Carb Cycle, you're going to be shocked how easy it is to actually unlock the fat burning potential of your body. My Carb Cycle is not complicated and best of all will never require you to go totally without carbs for any day or even meals like so many other diets unfortunately nowadays do. I've taught my specific diet approach to all kinds of people from all walks of life, and everyone catches on quickly and confirms how much sense this way of eating actually makes.

My book is really a fitness guide to life. In the first part, I explain what Carb Cycle is and why it works, and in the second part, I show you exactly how to do it. You'll only need to read the first part once to understand the concept and system. I'll also explain why other diets, cycles, and fitness programs do not have sustainable results and how the body's fat burning mechanism and its carb storage system interact. I will guide you one-on-one with food choices, meal plans, and the "right" carb cycle schedule - along with different fitness levels from beginner, to intermediate, to advanced, and much more. Most importantly, I will teach you to implement my Carb Cycle Method right away into your own, individual lifestyle. Then, once you achieved your new lean and healthy body, I will show you how to maintain it for life.

Once you learn and apply my Carb Cycle Method, you'll be able to melt the fat off your body and keep it off for good by EATING *THE RIGHT* CARBS ON JUST *THE RIGHT* CYCLE.

Maybe you want to lose a little extra weight to fit into a smaller size. Or maybe you want to get extra lean and toned up for that swimsuit, or even absolutely shredded for a fitness competition. Either way, my Carb Cycle Diet will give you the lean and healthy body you've always wanted and dreamed of and will enable you to keep it for life. Let's get started!

CHAPTER 1

THE ROAD TO
OPTIMUM FITNESS

MY PERSONAL PHILOSOPHY ON FITNESS

Achieving and maintaining top physical and mental shape is not only my profession, but also my passion. With persistence and healthy living, I have learned how to achieve peak physical and mental conditioning in a natural way, without any drugs, stimulants, or gimmicks. Taking stimulants or drugs to achieve top fitness has always been contrary to my personal code of ethics!

Unfortunately, there are too many unhealthy shortcuts and gimmicks available today. I realized early on that people who take shortcuts usually end up over the long-term not being in good shape and destroying their health. Because of this, I decided right at the beginning of my fitness career to stay healthy and reach my goals naturally. However, I was also determined to become world champion and to find a way to achieve top fitness as fast as possible, *AND* maintain it for the long term. This may have been an idealistic attitude of a naive teenager, but coupled with my passion I'm happy to report that over the years I have discovered and formulated a natural *AND* effective method to quickly get in great shape, and most importantly, how to stay that way. This method is the culmination of my twenty-seven plus years of studying, testing, and perfecting countless fitness techniques and routines.

The really good news is that you get the immediate benefits of my experience. **I've taken the guesswork out of dieting and fitness, and you will never have to go on another frustrating program again. I promise that if you apply my Carb Cycle System in your own life, you will see dramatic results quicker than you would have ever thought possible.**

MY JOURNEY TO MR. WORLD FITNESS

Growing up, my friends and I worshipped heroes like Superman, James Bond, and Rocky. They became our inspiration. However, while my friends merely dreamed of being strong like these super heroes, I went one step further. I went about strengthening my muscles in the real world. Then, one day I saw the former Mr. World, Steve Reeves, play the part of Hercules, and right away I knew what I wanted to be when I grew up. I remember begging my mother to let me stay up late so I could watch his movies. Then, I'd go to bed dreaming that one day my physique would resemble his. Now, I am in the same position, holding the title that he had the honour of holding five decades before me. For me, this has been a dream come true.

Growing up in Switzerland, I was fortunate to be able to take advantage of my amazing surroundings and find fantastic outlets for my athleticism. When I was about eleven years old, I knew I wanted to learn everything I could about health and fitness and my Birthday and Christmas wish lists became all about fitness books and dumbbells. Since I was too young to work out at the gym, these gifts allowed me to work out at home. Truth be told, I drove my mother a little crazy. I stopped eating the skin on the chicken, turned away sweets, and drank so much water that I'm surprised we had any left to wash the dishes. Out of what my family hoped was just a crazy stage, sprang a respect and love for fitness that continues today. For the record, my mother forgave me for driving her crazy all those years when she saw me win my Mr. World Titles, and more importantly, inspire people everywhere, including many of her friends, to become fit and healthy.

I entered my first competition at age 15 - Teenage Mr. Switzerland. If I had used the same diet and workout techniques that I used back then to compete in Mr. World Fitness, I would have surely lost. Back then, I didn't know how to diet and exercise the right way. In this competition, I ended up taking the kind, but misguided, suggestion of a gym owner who advised I go on a very low calorie, almost starvation diet. Looking back, this diet was the worst thing I could have done. That's because my metabolism simply collapsed and compensated for the nutritional deficit my diet created what actually kept me from getting into my best shape. Notwithstanding, I somehow ended up getting second place in that competition, and coming in second made me even more determined to work hard and learn more. As I look back, I realize how totally confused I was about dieting. Sadly, this confusion lasted for years.

Even with all the information I received from experts, trainers, friends, magazines, and books, I was constantly misinformed. I jumped from one diet to the next, one exercise program to the next: Low-carbs, no-carb, high-carbs, low-fat, high-intensity, low-intensity, and so on. It was very frustrating.

Still, I was determined to win the Mr. Teenage Switzerland title. I began to eat more frequently in order to keep my metabolism running efficiently. I also started to fine-tune my exercise routine and – what I luckily realized early on – focus on finding a way to eat carbs in exactly the right way. I just didn't give up and I ended up winning the competition. Although it took many more years for me to truly understand how my body worked, I knew I was on the right path.

I was fortunate enough to go on and win the IFBB (International Federation of Bodybuilding & Fitness) Mr. Switzerland title three times in a row. After that I moved on to competing internationally. Once again, after plenty of failures and mistakes, with various diets and exercise programs, I started to put the puzzle of optimal fitness together - piece by piece - and finally succeeded! After 15 years of searching for the best way to get in amazing shape, I finally became Mr. World Fitness for the first time.

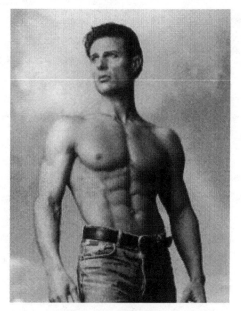

In peak Mr. World Fitness Shape

From my experiences I learned a number of things. First, doing a low-calorie or low-carb diet only made my metabolism slow down and this kept me from getting into my best shape. Second, there are many wrong ways, but only one right way to diet and exercise in order to achieve and maintain ultimate fitness. This took me many years to figure out. It was very frustrating but there just wasn't an accurate source of information I could draw from to help me get in perfect shape. However, as I persisted in my efforts, I figured out the things that worked, and what didn't. I continued down this path of refinement for many years and now have the answers to achieving the ultimate fitness level that most of us are looking for.

WHAT IS THE MR. WORLD FITNESS TITLE?

The judges in the Mr. World Fitness competition look for the person who embodies optimum, balanced fitness of both body and mind. The contestant who comes closest to an overall sculpted, toned and shaped body wins. Unlike bodybuilding, the "optimum" and not the "maximum" physical ideal is what matters in the final analysis, the way bodybuilding originally started in the 1940's.

Steve Reeves, the person I mentioned earlier, personified this ideal in the 1950's. It was also in the 50's when Sean Connery, the famous actor, competed in the NABBA Mr. World Competition. From the 70's on, hardcore bodybuilding began to totally take over the Mr. World title. The contestants became more and more massive, making it difficult for normal people to identify or associate with them anymore. In the 90's, the NABBA formed the World Fitness Federation (WFF) and shortly after the Mr. World competition was for the first time divided into two categories, Mr. World Bodybuilding and Mr. World Fitness. The WFF was the first Organization that started these kind of competitions. I was very fortunate to be at the right time at the right place all ready to claim this title after first competing for years in the IFBB, where I was a four time Mr. Switzerland, and then in the WNBF, a Natural Bodybuilding Organization - which included taking multiple drug tests along with a Polygraph (lie detector). Something I would gladly do anytime and anywhere to prove my 100% natural way of fitness. I won the Mr. World Fitness Title 6-times in a row and am proud to have been part of the History written at the beginning of the Men's Fitness Era. Meanwhile there are many other organizations that stepped in and started conducting fantastic Mr. and Miss Fitness competitions, although sometimes, the ideal fitness look lately almost too much tends to reflect the look of hard-core bodybuilding. That said, my preferred way of fitness will always be the optimally toned, lean, balanced, and not the maximally developed human body.

THE TRUTH ABOUT FITNESS

My first Mr. World Fitness win allowed me to really understand the essence of fitness. When I won I almost had to laugh because after years of frustration, I realized how easy it was to get in great shape. As soon as I learned the secret of how to cycle my carbs effectively and balance my diet and exercise routines, I knew the Mr. World Fitness title would be mine again, and again and again! And it was.

While I feel very blessed to hold all of my Mr. World Fitness titles, the greatest privilege for me is to share what I have learned and discovered with the world. Fortunately, before, during, and after my Mr. World Fitness Competitions, I wrote down all my techniques and concepts to achieve and maintain the greatest fitness possible. Now, it is my vision to inspire and educate an entire generation of people to achieve **THEIR** highest fitness, health, and wellness potential. To me, this is worth more than any title.

Once again, the great thing about this book is that you get the immediate benefits of all my years of research and experimentation. You no longer have to go on all those frustrating diets and exercise programs. I've already done it for you. I've taken the guesswork out of everything and now I can give you the benefit of my experience and the truth about fitness.

FITNESS, DIETING, AND CARBOHYDRATES: IT CAN BE TOTALLY CONFUSING

I am amazed after all my years in the industry how the business of fitness continues to grow. In the USA alone, billions of dollars are spent every year in the pursuit of fitness. Today, there are more diets, exercise books, videos, classes, trainers, fitness experts, and information available than ever before. However, at the same time, the majority of people I meet are totally confused, frustrated, and out of shape. In fact, at any given time, every third person is on a serious diet plan, yet more than two out of three adults are overweight and obese.

Why is this the case? I believe it's because even though we have so much information available, there still isn't a quality fitness system or way of fitness that provides **BOTH: RESULTS AND SIMPLICITY**.

To highlight this point, I recently went to a bookstore on a mission. I wanted to find one fitness book or system, which could illustrate clearly and safely how to get and stay in great shape. I spent half a day and didn't really find one that encompassed what I was looking for. Instead, I found dozens of books that were confusing, tedious, and potentially dangerous.

I'm sure you know exactly what I'm talking about. One book tells you not to eat carbohydrates at all, while the next one tells you to make them the foundation of your daily diet. The same misinformation abounds regarding eating fat, exercising, and every other aspect of diet and fitness. It's no wonder that people jump from one diet to the next, one exercise program to the next, only to end up disillusioned and still out of shape.

I promise that I will dispel the myths about fitness and give you the absolute truth. I'm not here to offer you overnight solutions or the promise that you'll have a six-pack within the next couple of days. However, I am here to give you a logical plan that's easy to understand and that really works and **WILL** get you there. Plus, I will reveal the secrets of how to jumpstart your weight loss goals with the most effective combination of diet and exercise around. I will show you how to get in the best shape of your life as fast as humanly possible. Even more important, I will show you how to maintain your newfound lean and healthy body forever and become fit for life!

Now, as we move forward, I want you to make a commitment to yourself and an investment in your fitness and well-being. The greatest gift that you can give yourself is that of a strong, healthy body and mind. Make the Carb Cycle which I often call the "**Cycle of Life**" your own lifestyle! I will show you how and after incorporating what I teach you, you won't believe the transformation your body will make.

So, if you're tired of being confused or out of shape, then get ready for a system that's simple to understand, easy to follow *AND* extremely effective. Together let's open the door to your optimum Fitness. Our journey will put you on the path to wellness, health, and happiness. Enjoy the ride because your life will never be the same!

CHAPTER 2

WHAT'S WRONG WITH THE TYPICAL DIET

WHY MOST DIETS DON'T WORK

Did you know there are over 17,500 published diets in the United States? You would think that with so many diets to choose from, every single person would find something that worked for them. Unfortunately, this isn't the case. Most people are so confused about dieting and how to lose weight, that rather than finding a plan that works, they jump from one diet to the next, only to experience frustration with their lack of results. In fact, most diets are so ineffective for people that two years after beginning a diet, and initially losing weight, 97% have either regained the weight they lost, or are heavier than when they first started dieting.

Most people quit dieting for two reasons. First, the majority of diets don't give you the results you're looking for; and second, most diets are designed to be too restrictive. They deprive your body from calories and nutrients, and as a result, your metabolism slows down to a point where it's practically impossible to lose weight.

So why do people have such a hard time with dieting? Well, anyone that has dieted, and that's mostly everyone, can probably answer this question. Diets fail for two reasons.

First, most people approach dieting like a sprint. All that matters are short-term results! After years of putting weight on, they go to drastic lengths to shed weight as fast as they possibly can. They do this by going on a diet that promises quick, but unsustainable results. As you probably know, these diets don't work and can't be maintained for the long-term. Plus, they often come with numerous negative side effects. Notwithstanding this, it doesn't stop people from constantly trying them.

The simple truth is that if you want to lose weight *AND* keep it off, then it's important to adopt eating changes that **can be sustained for a lifetime. Losing and maintaining weight should be considered more like a journey, instead of a sprint.** There's absolutely nothing wrong with following a diet that's designed to get you to your desired weight reasonably quickly, but only if the same diet also lets you maintain these results for the rest of your life. At the same time, any good diet won't slow down your metabolism or sacrifice your health and well-being. The trick to doing this is making the diet you follow so easy and logical, that it doesn't seem like a diet. And that's one of the greatest advantages of my Carb Cycle approach to eating. It's easy to do and it gets incredible *AND* sustainable results because it works exactly the way your body and its fat burning mechanism are made to function optimally.

The second reason diets fail is that people quit dieting. That's because the majority of diets are designed to be too restrictive. They are either **calorie restrictive** or **choice restrictive**, and both of these diets require a great deal of discipline to follow, especially if they require a total elimination of Carbs at any time of their program. Let me explain each of these diets:

14

CALORIE RESTRICTIVE DIETS

Calorie restrictive diets encourage eating very small amounts of food. These diets are often called "starvation" or "mouse diets". They are mostly based on eating fewer calories. The problem is that the body doesn't really think in terms of calories – but rather in terms of nutrients. One hundred calories from an apple isn't the same as a hundred calories coming from candy. These diets can be very dangerous to your health and should be avoided at all costs. They are very hard to follow and can cause a host of health problems. Although you may experience some weight loss in the short-term, it's usually just that – short term. Your body adjusts quickly to eating less food and this makes it almost impossible to lose more weight. These diets wreak havoc on a person's metabolism and health, and this is the last thing you want to do when trying to lose weight. (We'll talk more about metabolism later.)

Always remember that YOUR BODY DOESN'T "THINK" IN CALORIES, BUT IN NUTRIENTS! This is the reason why a lot of junk food can still leave you feeling hungry. Too-restrictive diets are never healthy either. Both approaches deprive your body of its vital nutrients.

CHOICE RESTRICTIVE DIETS

On the other hand, choice restrictive diets eliminate certain foods from your diet. A person following a choice restrictive diet typically over-eats certain kinds of foods and nutrients, while completely ignoring others. These extreme types of diets include things like constant low-carb or no-carb diets, low-fat diets, blood type diets, and so on. Unless there is a medical condition or allergy that requires you going on these types of diets, it's usually not a good idea.

Now, although both calorie and choice restrictive diets can make you lose weight in the short-term, they just don't work long-term. While cutting calories can help people lose weight, and most of us probably need to eat less than we currently do, any diet that promotes eating minimal amounts of food, or the same kinds of food, for a long period of time, doesn't typically work for the average person. If you've ever gone on a restrictive diet, then you know what I'm talking about. People just aren't designed to spend their lives eating tiny amounts of the same foods.

The good news is that my Carb Cycle Diet works both in the short-term and long-term. It doesn't restrict the amount or type of food you eat, and is the best diet ever created because it works with the way your body and its two energy storage systems (fat and carbs!) are made to function properly.

---

1) CALORIE RESTRICTIVE DIETS
Based on cutting calories to
extremely low levels.

2) CHOICE RESTRICTIVE DIETS
Based on eliminating certain
food groups from your diet.

Let's look closer at what's both good and bad about these two types of diets. We'll start by discussing calorie restrictive diets. Unfortunately, as you'll soon discover, these diets have a lot more "bad" than "good."

SOME EXAMPLES OF CALORIE RESTRICTIVE DIETS

Calorie restrictive diets include any diet that suggests to severely restrict the amount of food you eat. Let's take a look:

THE STARVATION OR MOUSE DIET

Starvation diets encourage people to eat well below what they should. When a person does this, they usually experience a quick drop in weight, but unfortunately, this initial drop in weight is only partly due to a loss of body fat. It's mostly water. After a short period of time, the weight loss slows down. In fact, it typically grinds to a halt. After all, there's only so much water your body can lose. At this point, the dieter gets frustrated by not seeing the results they once did. Adding to this, not eating an adequate amount of food has made them hungry, irritable, and lethargic.

Inevitably, most people who begin a starvation diet quickly return to eating their normal amount of food. This causes the "water weight" that so quickly came off, to quickly return. Any fat that they lost comes back too, and often times more than what they lost. Your body does this because it's on high-alert from being deprived of food. It doesn't want to get caught off guard and will store a little extra fat just in case you decide to starve yourself again in the future. What happens next is the really tragic part of what starvation diets can cause. In an effort to lose weight again, the dieter starves themselves once more, and then sees the same results. Sadly, this cycle repeats itself over and over. Losing and re-gaining weight like this is often referred to as a "yo-yo diet" or the "yo-yo effect," and there are a couple of serious consequences to doing this.

First, your greatest ally, or enemy, when trying to lose weight is your basal metabolic rate, or your metabolism. This is the rate at which your resting body burns calories. From a simple standpoint, the higher your metabolism the more food you can eat without putting on weight. Likewise, the lower your metabolism, the less food you can eat without putting on weight. You have probably seen this. Some people can eat whatever they want and not get fat, while others seems to put on weight by just looking at food?

So, if you're looking to lose weight, it should be your goal to increase your metabolism and there are certain ways to do this, but I can assure you, that starving yourself isn't one of them. When you consume fewer calories, your body adjusts its metabolic rate down. This means that your body acknowledges that it has to survive on fewer calories or nutrients, and slows down the rate at which it uses incoming energy. This translates into you not being able to eat as much food without putting on weight, as well as not being able to burn hardly any fat.

Second, a starvation diet wreaks havoc on your psychological well-being. When people resume eating after starving themselves, they tend to feel guilty for not demonstrating adequate self-control. Unfortunately, what many people don't know is that a starvation diet is almost impossible to stick to. Notwithstanding, this feeling of guilt usually lulls the person into beginning another starvation diet, and when this inevitable fails, the guilt returns. This constant cycle of feeling guilty and associating it with food can lead to some serious eating disorders that sometimes require professional help. Just another reason to avoid starvation diets at all costs.

Finally, although not exhaustive, the following list includes some of the problems that can arise from starvation dieting. We've already discussed how these diets lower your metabolic rate (metabolism) and how they can lead to eating disorders. However, they can also lead to joint pain, hair loss, muscle loss, osteoporosis, depression, lack of energy, insomnia, moodiness, bad breath, and decreased sexual desire.

The bottom line is that if you are trying to lose weight, it's really important that you don't try doing it by going on a starvation type diet. Granted, most people probably need to eat less than they do, but going to the extreme and hardly eating anything isn't the answer. If you're on one of these diets, then please stop. I will show you a better way that I promise will give you the results you're looking for, without any of the negative side effects.

Although my Carb Cycle Diet doesn't require you to count calories, the average man should never eat less than 1,300-1,800 calories per day, and the average woman should never eat less than 1,200-1,500 calories per day. You should further adjust these numbers based on your activity levels.

SOME EXAMPLES OF CHOICE RESTRICTIVE DIETS

Choice restrictive diets include any diet that limits or cuts certain foods out completely, favors one food over another, or fails to recommend the appropriate balance of carbs, fats, and proteins.

Let's look at a few of these diets and analyze how they work:

THE LOW AND NO-CARB DIETS

Any extremely low or no-carb diets fall into the choice restrictive category as they are based on eating little to virtually no carbohydrates, sometimes even constantly. These diets often don't even allow you to eat healthy grains, fruits, or vegetables for whole days or eliminate them altogether, which just doesn't make any sense at all.

So what's the theory behind these kinds of diets? Why would someone want to deprive themselves of eating any carbs at all?

Well, when someone doesn't eat carbs for a certain period of time, they go into a state called ketosis. Ketosis is a process whereby a person's body is directed to use fat and protein reserves as a source of energy, because all the carb reserves are gone. Depending on your personal activity and restriction level of carb intake, your body can rid itself of carbs within 1-3 days, and it is *DURING* this initial carb-draining phase that the low-carb diet actually works wonders. Here's why:

Carbs are one of your body's primary sources of energy. When carbs are restricted from your diet, your body quickly looks to other fuel sources for energy, primarily fat. It is during this carb draining phase where you can experience substantial fat burn and weight loss without jeopardizing your metabolism.

Unfortunately though, the initial results from following a low-carb or no-carb diet never last. After a few days, your body will reach ketosis (the state of an empty carb storage), or be very close to it, and will adapt to being with little or no carbs. This will cause your metabolism to slow down and that's when losing additional weight becomes very difficult. You may have noticed this with people who are on a constant low-carb diet. You may have even experienced it yourself. Even worse: being on a complete "no-carb" diet, even for only 1 or 2 meals in a row, puts your body on high-alert immediately and potentially slows down your metabolism within hours.

One of the great things about my Carb Cycle program is that it provides all the advantages of going low-carb or no-carb, but not just for some hours or one day. Your results won't plateau, you won't get irritable, and you can still eat all of your favorite carbs on a regular basis without feeling guilty.

Although your body can survive without eating carbs, being on a constant low-carb diet, or even worse an absolute "no-carb" diet, can have many downsides. These include:

- Decreased metabolism
- Depression
- Increased irritability
- Loss of concentration
- Loss of energy
- Loss of strength
- High cholesterol
- Lack of fiber
- Vitamin deficiencies
- Dehydration
- Gastrointestinal problems
- Low Libido
- Kidney disease
- Gallbladder disease, and
- Heart disease

Also, if you have an active lifestyle or want to become more active, don't even think about starting a constant low-carb diet or no-carb diet. You simply won't have enough energy to function properly. Carbs give energy and you can't exercise if you don't have any energy.

The bottom line is that living with very low, or even no carbs, is not a viable option for losing weight and keeping it off. Carbs are essential for your body to operate properly. While it makes sense to temporarily drain your carbohydrate reserves slowly, there's just no rational reason to stay this way. As discussed above, once the initial draining phase of a low-carb diet is complete, your energy will drop and losing any more weight becomes very difficult. Plus, many low-carb diets often encourage to balance out this deficiency of carbs and energy by eating more (sometimes even unhealthy, saturated!) fat choices, which aren't really good for your body either.

Your basal metabolic rate, or the amount of energy you simply need to stay alive, can account for as much as 70% of the calories you burn. This is why it's never a good idea to slow that 24/7 Power Machine down, especially if you want to keep losing weight in the long haul and feel energetic & great while doing so!

THE NO FAT, HIGH-CARB DIETS

Talk about the opposite of the low-carb approach. The goal of the no-fat, high-carb diets is to avoid fat at all cost, while eating almost as much carbs as you want. Constantly eating a lot of Carbs while keeping them "lean" was very popular in the 80's and early 90's, just before Atkins, who became famous as the initiator of the low and no-carb diets. Lately, there are many diets that suggest to go back to this approach, fueled by "low-carb tired" dieters who desperately search for a way to eat carbs again. People following this approach believe eating carbs while eliminating fat is the best way to stay fit and healthy. This thinking stems from years of being brainwashed by "experts" that suggest all fats are bad, and all carbs are good. But what's the truth? Well, it is somewhere in the middle, in fact both Atkins and Carb Lovers have it "half right"!

Simply cutting fat from your diet is not an effective way to lose weight. In fact, doing this can actually make your body crave fat and consequently, hold on to it. Plus, there are certain fats that are essential to healthy living. These include monounsaturated fats and omega-3 fats. These are found in things like vegetable oils, nuts, seeds, avocados, and fish, and are suggested to be pivotal in preventing heart disease, cancer and many other diseases. Your body needs these types of fat in moderation every day, even if your goal is to actually lose fat. With that said though, not all fats are good. Bad fats, especially saturated fats are found in animal products such as beef, pork, and lamb. Saturated fats also include dairy products such as cheese and butter. As well as having to worry about saturated fats, perhaps of even more concern are trans fatty acids. These are created during certain cooking procedures and are found in things like candy, cakes, deep fried foods, pastries, etc. Consuming large quantities of trans fatty acids have been linked to an increase in the risk of several chronic diseases. Limiting these fats in your diet is certainly a good idea.

On the flip side, eating large or even normal quantities of carbs all the time comes with its own set of problems too. That's because under certain circumstances, carbs can be converted into fat. This happens when your body's natural carb storage areas, your muscles and liver, are full. Whenever these areas are full, the carbs you eat get turned into fat.

The secret to eating carbs and not having them turn to fat is knowing when to eat exactly what kind of carbs, and that is something I will teach you. Unfortunately though, most people have no clue as to how to do this and that makes the no-fat/high-carb diet a very bad choice for losing weight.

It is very amusing to me that most diet experts have no clue how to set up an exercise program. Plus, many times the people who invent diets aren't in great shape. How can a diet possibly work if the expert who represents it is NOT in great shape himself? Even worse, what if they are but achieved their results by doing other things like drugs?

EXOTIC DIETS:
THE "ZONE", BLOOD-TYPE, SOUTH BEACH DIETS, ETC.

There are many diets that suggest you eat by color or by your blood type, or some other fancy way. No matter what it is, these diets are either too flexible by suggesting you eat according to how you feel, or they're too restrictive by allowing you to only eat certain foods. Whatever the case, as we've discussed, choice restrictive diets rarely work over the long term.

So what's wrong with these exotic diets? Well, they often make you avoid foods that are perfectly healthy to eat in a balanced way. For example, many of these diets tell you to avoid foods like potatoes, rice, cereal, and bread. However, cutting these foods out of your diet is no guarantee that you'll lose weight. Other exotic diets tell you to be cautious with foods like whole grains, fruits, starches, and vegetables. In my opinion, if eaten in moderation and as part of the right diet system, these foods are a perfectly fine component of any healthy way of eating.

The bottom line is that exotic diets don't work very well because most times they lack common sense. Many of these fancy or restrictive diets are limiting and therefore work on a limited basis. When it comes to choosing a diet, you need to be logical and stick with the basics of nutrition. Also, remember to use your intuition and common sense. If you don't understand a diet and how it works, then be cautious. Just using a little common sense will cause you to avoid the wrong kinds of foods and diets. In closing, some of these "exotic diets" are not necessarily bad for you and can give you some results, but there is a better way if you want to eat all kind of foods you love *AND* get and stay in great shape most effectively!

THE CARB "THIS" OR CARB "THAT" DIETS

Since I developed and perfected my Carb Cycle Diet in the 90's there have been a lot of diets, especially recently, that make claims or promises with names and titles such as "Carb Solution" or "Carb Secret". Some of them even started using the word "Cycle" or "Cycling" in one way or another. However, when closely looking at these diets, **none of them mention or work with the human body's carb storage system in the natural, proper, and most efficient way I'm going to present in this book** (*Note: You might want to re-read this section after completing the book to understand it even better*). In the best cases, they either tell you to go **low-carb for too short lengths of time,** sometimes only for parts of the day or one day, or they tell you to go **low-carb for more than 2-3 days** which puts you on an empty carb storage for too long again. Further, they do not teach you **which carbs exactly to cycle,** but just **cut all carbs out equally.** Even worse, some new diets suggest to go **"no-carb" which you should never do, not even for a single day or meal**, except maybe the last meal of the day after 6pm! As you will learn in this book, and what took me 27 years to fine-tune, the **most effective carb cycle is when you empty and fill your storage "as slowly as possible" in order to** maximize fat-burning and prevent your body from "panic-ing" and shutting down its metabolism. Ideally, depleting your body's carbs will take 2-3 days and **can be achieved without ever going completely without carbs**. Loading carbs can always be achieved much faster since the body stores carbs quicker than it burns them off. Therefore, any real "efficient" carb cycle always has more "low-carb" days than high-carb days. It's like a cell phone battery, loading it goes much faster than draining it - if done correctly. At the same time, super-draining doesn't make sense with a cell phone battery and it doesn't make sense with your body's carb storage either. That's why **carb diets or cycles that tell you to go completely without carbs are just not ideal, even if it's just for one meal or day.**

Having talked about too little or no carbs, on the contrary, some of the same diets tell you to eat more carbs or even especially **high amounts of carbs for more than 1-2 days or even whole weeks** as a regular part of their "diet" or "cycle" which puts you in the situation of having a full, or even worse, overfilled carb storage system for many days, weeks, or even months. Keep reading this book and you'll learn for yourself why this never makes sense either. You will realize soon that most diets just use the name "Carb" or "Cycle" as a catchy add on but when you look closely at them, they are just another variation of a moderation diet, or food or choice restrictive diet. Some of them **lately do actually somehow cycle carbs - but in the "wrong" cycle and intensity** as I just explained. For example, a very common technique recently is to **go high or normal-carb for one day followed by a single low or - what you should *NEVER* do - even no-carb day**. That is not really a practical or rational Cycle, but more of a **rushed & extreme "draining and loading" practice**. The only ones who can – or must - do this are extreme athletes such as cyclists who drain their carbs in a single day or even just some hours because they ride their bikes for long periods of time. Something by the way they could never keep on doing for longer than 1-2 weeks.

However, for **optimum fat-burning it's important to "drain" the body's carb storage system "as slowly and steadily" as possible over 2-3 days** in order to burn a maximum amount of fat and - **most importantly** - *NEVER completely go without carbs, not even for any daily meals.* Carbs are integral in so many body functions and even a single meal or day **where "carbs are not an option" period can potentially have many unwanted and unnecessary side effects.** Additionally, some diets using their ""ineffective" carb cycles not only cut out carbs completely, **but also vegetables or other basic food groups such as milk products.** This is going against any common sense as well as **Worldwide Governmental Guidelines which all recommend eating at least 5 fruits and vegetables daily.** I couldn't agree more with this, and whenever you hear about other diets that might look or sound interesting but lack common sense or authenticity: be careful. Especially in case they become too restrictive, cut all carbs out, or are just too intense to follow in the long term like all the kind of diets I just discussed in this chapter.

In conclusion, to be fair to other carb diets and cycles, most of these diets and systems **are rather new and based on good intentions to help people lose weight.** But they **are just not based on many years of experience. In fact it took me over 20 years of constant fine-tuning until I formulated the most efficient Carb Cycle Method I'll teach you in this book.**

Any "new" diet that uses a Carb "X" title but keeps you on either low, no, or high-carb for either too few or too many days in a row doesn't consider or take advantage of the Human Body's Carb Storage System in the correct way. Keep reading this book and learn why there is only one real and effective way of Carb Cycle. Soon you will be a "detector" of any other ineffective diet system out there, and will instantly know the pros and cons!

CONCLUSION: WHAT'S THE BEST COMMON SENSE DIET?

Calorie and choice restrictive diets aren't the perfect answer. Low-Carb for too long or Normal-Carb all the time isn't either. Cutting carbs completely out for even a single meal is definitely not the answer. But what is? What kind of eating plan will allow you to be successful in losing weight and keeping it off for good *while* feeling great and having more energy?

First, as strange it might sound, you need to **stop traditional dieting by thinking of a diet as a quick fix solution to losing weight. A good diet is a way of eating, not just a way to lose weight, and certainly not a temporary phase where you should suffer**. If you really want to lose weight and keep it off for good, you have to adopt a healthy, logical approach towards your body and food. **Eating right is a journey and not a sprint.** A good diet will allow you to lose weight as fast as possible *AND* maintain that success in the long-term as well. The only eating plan that a person will stay on long-term is one that is easy to follow. Within reason, a diet shouldn't restrict the amount or choice of food that you eat. If you're considering starting any diet, always ask yourself, "Can I stay on this diet forever?" If your answer is no, don't start this type of diet. Instead, look for a diet that you know you can maintain over the long term for life.

Second, a diet should be **logical, simple to understand and implement.** It should be based on **a balance of all available healthy food choices,** as well as acknowledging the **Body's Natural Carb Cycle Storage System.** It should include regular amounts of good quality protein and healthy fat choices, along with a sensible approach towards carbohydrates. It should allow you to eat any kind of healthy, natural food. It should also include regular days where you can cheat and eat all kinds of food. After all, we're only human. Finally, a good diet should allow you to control whether you want to maintain or lose weight. It should also work without exercising, but still it should be possible to combine it with any exercise program in order to enhance results. Adding regular exercise is always the healthier, better option.

So, taking these points into consideration, what is the best diet? It's my Carb Cycle Diet of course. Any diet that doesn't respect, or ignores your ability to store and burn carbs in the correct, most efficient, and healthiest cycle is incomplete and limits your results. And that's exactly what we're going to discuss in the next couple of chapters.

CHAPTER 3

THE TRUTH
ABOUT CARBS

In the Seventies and Eighties there was a "High-Carb Mania," where the popular diets of the day recommended eating large amounts of carbohydrates. Then, in the nineties until today, the opposite became more popular. Nowadays people everywhere seem to be avoiding carbs. In fact, this "low-carb mania" has swept the world and created legions of low-carb fanatics. Still, most of these people have no clue how their body uses carbs and how a certain carb lifestyle can either help them lose weight or totally destroy their goals and dreams. **So, once and for all, let me now explain what carbs are, how they work, and why you actually need them ALL THE TIME!**

YOUR BODY NEEDS CARBS!

Carbs, or carbohydrates, are forms of sugars. They act as the main source of fuel for your body and are necessary for you to function properly. In fact, they are the preferred food for your brain. The saying, "good food equals good mood", is by no means a myth. Your brain recognizes when you've eaten good food, especially good carbs. Good carbs usually come in natural, nutrient loaded foods like whole grains, beans, fruits, and vegetables. Plus, these foods contain lots of vitamins, minerals, and fiber. So with so much that is good about carbs, why do they have such a bad reputation?

NOT ALL CARBS ARE CREATED EQUAL

Although some carbs are beneficial to your health, others are not. In fact, most of the refined and highly processed foods, that have unfortunately become staples in our modern diets, are the kinds of carbs you should avoid. That's because our bodies were never designed to handle all these simple sugars and unhealthy additives we put in our food today. For example, **200 years ago the average "pure" sugar intake per person was less than 20 pounds per year. Now it's an estimated 200 pounds annually!** The reason: the invention of sugary foods and drinks. No wonder diabetes and other diseases are so common today, even in children.

Knowing the difference between "good" and "bad" carbs is important to any healthy living and weight control program, including the Carb Cycle. It's even more important to know how these carbs interact with the body's carb storage system and we will go over this very soon. However for now, discussing a few general carb related concepts will allow you to better understand more about carbs and how to best eat them. It will optimally prepare you for understanding my Carb Cycle Diet even better.

THE ROLE OF INSULIN

Although most people have heard of insulin, not many understand what it is or what it does. Simply stated, insulin is a naturally occurring hormone that's helps decrease and control a person's blood sugar levels. Here's how it works:

When you eat carbs your blood sugar level tends to go up. This makes sense since as we just mentioned, carbs are a form of sugar. Now, when this happens because your body doesn't like having your blood sugar levels outside of a normal range it responds by releasing insulin. The job of insulin is to then transport the sugar out of your bloodstream and into cells throughout your body. Doing this helps bring your blood sugar levels back to normal.

But where do the carbs, or sugars go? Well, they first look to go to cells in your muscles and your liver, but if that storage area is full, then excess carbs are transported to your fat cells. Once in your fat cells, these carbs are quickly converted into fat, and unfortunately, your fat cells are very greedy. Unlike your muscles and your liver, there is not really any limit to how much fat cells can convert and store. That's one of the reasons that people who consume a lot of sugar or a lot of carbs in general tend to become overweight or obese.

Even worse, the conversion of sugar to fat can happen almost instantaneously. Your body doesn't wait until the end of the day to do the math on what you've eaten and how much you've exercised. Instead, under certain circumstances sugar converts to fat very quickly. Fortunately, there are ways to virtually guarantee that the carbs you eat never get converted into fat. One way is to eat good quality carbs that release less insulin. Another way is to never overfill your natural carb storage areas, but instead slowly deplete and re-load them in an ongoing cycle. This is the basis of my Carb Cycle Diet and something we'll discuss more soon.

So what determines a "Good-Carb" from a "Bad-Carb"? One of the biggest differences in carbs is the **rate** at which they secrete insulin. For example, the carbs in a candy bar will produce a much greater amount of insulin, than the carbs in a vegetable. So, when it comes to losing weight and eating carbs, you should choose carbs that cause as little insulin secretion as possible. To help you make these better choices, carbs are scientifically ranked according to the rate in which they promote insulin secretion. This ranking system is known as the Glycemic Index. Let's talk more about it.

THE GLYCEMIC INDEX

The Glycemic Index Value is a measure of how much food affects insulin secretion. The higher the Glycemic Index of a food, the more it promotes the secretion of insulin. As discussed, there is a direct relationship between insulin production and weight gain.

As a rule of thumb, glycemic values mostly apply to carbs. So, in trying to control your weight, you should try to eat carbs that have a relatively low Glycemic Index Value. In order to do this you obviously need to know the glycemic values for carbs. However, instead of having to refer to the glycemic chart every time you want to eat carbs, let me show you how to easily figure out the difference between good and bad carbs.

THE 2 KINDS OF CARBS

Carbs can be defined as either complex or simple. They are defined this way based on their molecular structure. Let's look at both of them briefly:

SIMPLE CARBS

You can typically associate simple carbs with food that is refined, processed, and unnatural. These carbs have a high Glycemic Index Value and when eaten, they rapidly increase your blood sugar levels. Simple carbs are often called empty carbs or unhealthy carbs, as they are typically void of nutrients like fiber and vitamins.

Simple Carbs include Foods like:

- White Sugar
- Candy
- Soft Drinks
- Highly processed white Breads
- General baked Goods
- Sugary Cereals
- Exotic Fruits (containing more fruit sugar)

Simple Carbs should be avoided except on cheating days and meals. If eaten, they should be eaten when your carb storages areas are low or empty, never when they're full.

COMPLEX CARBS

On the other hand, complex carbs are typically unrefined, unprocessed, and natural. They have a relatively low Glycemic Index value as they come with lots of nutrients and fiber. They are digested more slowly and they don't promote the spike in insulin production like simple carbs do. They are therefore often referred to as "good carbs" or healthy carbs. These carbs are the best to eat, as they're less likely to be converted into fat. That is if they're eaten when your carb storage areas aren't full. (We'll talk more about this later.)

Complex Carbs include Foods like:

- Whole-Grain Pasta
- Brown Rice
- Oatmeal
- Potatoes
- Whole-Grain Products

- High fiber, sugar-free Cereals
- Vegetables and Legumes
- Northern Fruits (containing less fruit sugar)

Complex carbs are the carbs that should be preferred, except when there's a clear reason or you are on a cheat day. Good carbs are the foundation of any good diet.

THE INSULIN ROLLERCOASTER

Whenever you eat high Glycemic Index foods, like simple carbs, your body releases insulin quickly and in greater amounts to bring your blood sugar levels back to normal. When insulin levels rise too fast, you're potentially opening a door to fat storage, especially if your liver and muscle storage areas are full. Even worse, you will be hungry again in no time. That's because if blood sugar levels rise too fast, the body releases more insulin than it actually would take to stabilize your blood sugar level, so to say going from too-high to too-low, what is called "Rollercoaster". As your blood sugar level drops below that ideal zone, you'll feel tired and hungry again soon. This causes you to want to eat again, and under these circumstances, many times we tend to eat something "sugary". Doing this simply causes more than actually necessary insulin to be released again and pretty soon you're on an ongoing insulin rollercoaster. Besides that this feels very bad by making you moody and draining your energy, it also promotes the risk of type 2 diabetes.

Ideally, you should look to eat foods that keep your blood sugar levels relatively constant. This way insulin is released gradually (more slowly but steadily) into your bloodstream, giving you more energy and regulating your appetite. Plus, keeping your blood sugar level stable helps to prevent sugar from being converted into fat, especially if you never overfill your carb storage areas.

A WORD ON STARCHES, GRAINS, AND WHEAT

Carbohydrates also include starches, wheat, and other grains. These are foods like certain breads, potatoes, white rice, and pasta. Unfortunately, there are many experts telling you to avoid these foods completely. But what should you do?

Well, the truth is again somewhere in the middle. All natural foods, such as whole grains, potatoes, fruits, and vegetables are basically healthy food choices. The only thing to keep in mind is to eat them wisely and in the right amount. If you over eat any food, and most of us do, it will always lead to weight gain and/or digestion issues. But since Starches, Grains, and Wheat are natural foods, they're usually high in fiber and low in sugar and fat, so you shouldn't cut them totally out, unless of course you are allergic to them or have a medical condition.

For example, a potato, although starchy, is still a good source of fiber. It contains about 25% of your daily potassium along with calcium, vitamin C, and other minerals, especially if eaten with the peel. There's nothing wrong with eating potatoes, but in moderation and as part of a balanced diet. The same applies for bread or cereal. Just make sure that it's very low or free of sugar and made from grains. And don't forget to eat it based on whatever your Carb Cycle plan for the day is, something I will teach you soon.

Also, allow me to share a secret tip with you. There is a simple way that allows you to slow down the absorption of starchy carbohydrates like white rice or potatoes: eat them in combination with something that contains a good amount of fiber. For example, whenever I eat white rice or potatoes, I make sure to add some extra greens and vegetables, or consume a fiber drink at the same time. This will slow down the otherwise faster absorption of those starchy carbs. Whole grain products such as brown rice are always the better choice of course.

If you are concerned as many are nowadays about gluten - go to your doctor and do a test to find out if you are allergic. Most people are not allergic, that doesn't necessarily mean that gluten-free products are a bad choice. I personally like them and eat them on a regular basis. I would even agree that too many wheat and grain products which usually contain gluten are not the best choice. But as long as you eat them in moderation and cycle your carbs accordingly it can't really do much harm. By the way, did you ever ask yourself what the difference is between grain and wheat? Very simple: every wheat is a grain - but not every grain is a wheat! Barley, oats, or rye for example are a grain, but not a wheat. When it comes to gluten, it's even more complex and experts are debating the topic constantly. Thanks to Wikipedia you can look up the latest studies and news in more detail anytime if this interests you further.

But before you drive yourself crazy, my take home message here is don't let anybody make you believe that natural, healthy carbs make you fat, especially if you love to eat them. In fact "not" eating carbs at all with your daily meals or only in very small amounts all the time is even worse, something I will explain next! People get fat by eating carbs because they either over-eat carbs, or they eat the wrong ones at the wrong times. Even processed carbs can be part of a healthy diet plan, so long as you eat them wisely and at the right times.

Now that you've learned a little more about the quality of carbs, it's time to teach you the ins and outs about my Carb Cycle System.

CHAPTER 4

THE CARB CYCLE
SYSTEM

Unlike a traditional low-carb or no-carb diet that severely restricts carb consumption, my Carb Cycle Diet encourages eating carbs regularly as part of a (R)Evolutionary new approach. However, the manner in which you eat these carbs is what makes my Carb Cycle so unique and effective. Simply put, my Carb Cycle program re-arranges the way you eat certain carbs. It's a unique process where you eat carbs in a normal manner on specific days, while restricting certain carbs on other days.

If done correctly, this unique "Cycle" approach to eating carbs is a very powerful weight loss *AND* control technique as it allows you to eat carbs, naturally store them, and then very slowly burn them off. During this Carb Cycle process, your body burns fat faster and better than ever before. Best of all, compared to other diets and other "Cycles", my Carb Cycle never requires you to go completely without carbs which makes it much more doable as well as prolongs the fat-burning period to its maximum potential. All while keeping your energy levels high and never slowing own your metabolism.

Now, understanding how my Carb Cycle works requires a brief discussion on how our bodies are built to function, how and where they store energy, and why this affects the way we gain or lose weight.

THE CYCLE OF LIFE: UNDERSTANDING OUR PAST TO ACHIEVE SUCCESS TODAY

Out of necessity, our ancestors walked and hunted every day. They lived by a simple law created by Mother Nature: the law of balance between **1) eating food, 2) storing it,** and **3) burning it off** again. Here's what I mean by that. Activity was necessary to find food. Food provides energy, and this energy is used to function properly and find food again. This food, or energy, is stored by our bodies to be burned off when it's needed. This cycle repeats itself over and over.

If you look at wild animals, you see that they still follow this cycle. They have to be active in order to survive. That's why you'll never see a wild animal that is fat or out of shape. They are on the "Cycle of Life". The same Cycle that we used to follow. Well, not anymore.

Today, we can find food everywhere and eat it at any time. We don't have to hunt or forage for our food. Even worse, we have exponentially increased the amount of food we eat, all while decreasing the quality of it. Furthermore, because we have taken activity out of finding food, we are overloading our fat storage and do not empty and cycle our natural carb storage areas frequently enough which would prevent us from getting fat. But what exactly are these carb storage areas?

By using the principles of my Carb Cycle Diet, you can create and maintain results just like our forefathers who had to use their carb storage constantly in an "ongoing slow cycle" in order to survive.

Something that most people don't know and I mentioned many times already is that the human body actually has a "Carb Storage System". YES – YOU HAVE THE ABILITY TO STORE BOTH: FAT AND CARBOHYDRATES! While the body can store nearly an unlimited amount of fat in fat cells, it stores a limited amount of carbs in the muscles and the liver. Once these storage areas are full, any excess carbs you eat will be converted to fat. But why does our body do this?

As discussed above, our ancestors had to be active in order to eat. Sometimes it was difficult to find food every day. So, in order to help us survive during times when food was scarce for many days, our body would do two things. First, it would tap the naturally occurring fat and carb storage areas for energy. The second thing our body would do in times of scarce food is slow down an individual's metabolism as soon as the initial short-term carb storage was emptied. This mechanism was giving us the ability to survive on fewer calories. Now while this is great if you're trying to preserve energy until your next meal comes along, it isn't good if you're trying to lose weight.

This is why the body stores fat in an unlimited amount. It was for those times when food wasn't available, which of course doesn't really apply today. So how does knowing this help us today?

THE HUMAN BODY HAS BOTH: A FAT AND CARB STORAGE SYSTEM! Wouldn't it be great if our bodies realized that times had changed and just flushed any excess fat and carbohydrates that we eat? Unfortunately, that's not the way it works. To make it even worse, we eat so much processed, unhealthy food, that it just compounds the problem.

When we were forced to find our own food, our bodies didn't waste anything. This survival mechanism was great then, but not as helpful today. The regular cycle where our ancestors went with less or even without food, and were forced to tap or drain their natural carb storage areas, has a really amazing side effect: It burns fat like crazy! However, unlike our ancestors, you won't have to go without food to accomplish the same purpose. You can do it with my Carb Cycle Diet because I will teach you how. I'll also show you exactly when to eat what carbs without feeling guilty, and then how to flush them from your body to burn fat like never before. The bottom line is that our fat and carb storage systems are here whether we like them or not – so we might as well use them to our advantage.

Again, when your natural carb storage areas are full, any excess carbs you eat will be converted into fat. Sadly, most people's diets are either so carb depleted that it slows their metabolism down to a halt, or so carb-rich that their natural carb storage systems are almost always full. That's why nearly 100% of the carbs they eat go right to their fat cells. Neither situation is beneficial. There is a reason we have our storage systems. In the past we were always more or less on a Carb Cycle. Further, we ate all natural foods. Although times changed, these two rules stay the same.

CARB CYCLE: REDISCOVERING THE BODY'S CARB STORAGE SYSTEM

As mentioned above, most people don't know their bodies have a natural storage mechanism for both fat and carbs. The fat gets stored in fat cells, and carbs in your muscles and liver. Actually, the carbs you eat are converted to glucose and are stored as glycogen. However, we will refer to stored glycogen as stored carbs.

Also, while you have an almost unlimited capacity to store fat, there is a limit to the amount of carbs you can store. Once these reserves are full, incoming carbs are directed to your fat cells. Fat cells are more like a secondary, "extra" storage, while carbs are ideally the main energy source and preferred storage of your body. Obviously, if you're trying to lose or maintain weight, you'd for sure rather carbs be deposited into your liver and muscles instead of your fat cells. How is this accomplished though?

The answer is very simple: **using the Body's Carb Storage System "again" to its full capacity with the only efficient and most effective the Carb Cycle I teach you in this book!** Incoming carbs won't go to your fat cells if you eat them when your carb reserves aren't full. Your body always prefers to store carbs in your liver and muscles, not your fat cells. If you eat carbs when these reserves aren't at full capacity, then these carbs don't make it to your fat cells. However, if your natural carb reserves are full, then your body has no choice but to direct further carbs to your fat cells. **On the other side, always keeping your carb reserves low or empty, or depleting them too fast by eating no carbs at all, makes your metabolism and energy slow down, as well deprives you from certain nutrients. Most important, it prevents your body from experiencing the powerful fat burning process that happens when you're constantly and _VERY, VERY SLOWLY_ depleting and loading your carbs using an ongoing cycle.**

Although it depends on your individual size, on average your liver holds about 70-100 grams of carbs, and your muscles hold about 200-300 grams of carbs.

Think of it like this. Let's compare your natural carb storage system to a glass of water. Obviously, there's a limited amount of water that a glass can hold. If you add water to an already full glass, the water overflows. If the glass isn't full then adding more water simply fills up the glass. Only when the glass is full, will the water overflow. Also, if you put the water in too fast, it can spill over as well.

It's much the same with your natural carb storage areas, your liver and your muscles. They can only hold a certain amount in the way of carbs. If you keep eating carbs when these storage areas are at "carb capacity", these carbs will have no other choice than to be directed to your fat cells.

In relation to my Carb Cycle System, your goal is to start intentionally filling and emptying "your glass," especially if you want to burn fat and lose weight. Plus, you should ideally first deplete "your glass" as steadily and slowly as possible. Once it's empty or close to it, you want to fill it again slowly, by eating good quality carbs, instead of quickly by eating simple sugars. That way very few or no carbs will ever be converted into fat, and even better: **your body stays in a permanent Fat-Burning Zone!**

To give you another example, think about your cell phone. Aren't you constantly charging and draining the battery? Your carb storage is designed to do the same thing. To first store carbs, then drain them, and then store them again. Just keep in mind that you should never overload your storage system, or stay empty for too long. Further, rushing the whole process by cutting out carbs completely doesn't make sense either, because you would only put your body in high-alert and instantly shut its metabolism and fat-burning power down. **Remember: your body *ALWAYS* knows exactly what's going on and adjusts very quickly.**

THE PERFECT DIET FOR EVERYONE

If carbs don't have the chance to reach your fat cells then it's pretty hard to get fat from eating carbs - isn't it?

The problem is that many people's diets are so carb-concentrated that their carb reserves are usually always full, and almost all of the carbs they eat get directed to their fat cells. On the other extreme, constant low or no-carb diets keep us in a state where our natural carb reserves are almost always empty. These diets slow down your metabolism and leave you with low energy, making the body preserve fat instead of releasing it. Remember, that was the mechanism that kept our ancestors alive but it doesn't work to your advantage today because food is so readily available.

When it comes to Dieting and Carbs, the Metabolism slows down whenever the following 2 Scenarios occur: 1) a constant low-carb status which results in a constant low-carb storage, or 2) any "total" elimination of carbs, even if it's for just one or two daily meals. These tactics put the body into high-alert and instantly make him preserve energy and slow down its basal metabolic rate, thereby blocking any optimum fat-burning and weight-loss results, especially in the long-term.

To combat both of those problems, my Carb Cycle Diet encourages you periodically to slowly drain your carb reserves for 2-3 days and then to eat carbs normally again for 1-2 days. When you do, they'll be directed to your body's natural carb reserves and not your fat cells, while your body happily burns down its fat storages at the same time. Your carb reserves are usually drained in two ways and we'll discuss that soon. Before we do this, let me explain more about the only kind of Carb Cycle Schedule that makes sense, and show you how easy it is to incorporate into your regular weekly schedule.

THE CARB CYCLE SCHEDULE

The process of my Carb Cycle Diet involves alternating the days whereby you eat and then restrict certain carbs. This routine allows you to drain your carb reserves slowly on certain days, and reload them on others. This slow and steady "drain-reload" process burns fat like nothing I've ever seen and is important for a few reasons:

1) **After slowly and steadily draining your body of its carb reserves, you can eat carbs with the assurance that these carbs won't be converted into fat.**

2) **Following my Carb Cycle program further enhances weight loss by encouraging you to eat the right kinds of foods, especially the right kinds of carbs, and**

3) **On the days where you "slowly and steadily" reduce your intake of certain carbs you will unlock the fat burning power of your metabolism. Re-loading carbs frequently in turn makes sure your metabolism never slows down but runs high 24/7.**

The reason you burn fat so quickly and efficiently during the draining phase of my program is that when you start to restrict the right carbs from your diet **slowly,** your body recognizes this and tries to preserve them for as long as possible. So while you're **slowly and steadily** depleting your carb reserves, **your body is willing to work with you instead of against you,** telling your fat cells to release as much fat as possible. It does this in order to protect its current carb storage for as long as possible. This is why it ideally takes 2-3 days to really empty your carb storage, because you are burning fat, and lots of it, at the same time. In fact, this is where you burn the most fat – the depleting stage. Once your storage areas are empty, the fat burning slows because the body realizes it ran out of carbs and slows down its metabolism. That's why you should never stay on a low-carb diet for long periods of time or even worse go on a diet that includes total carb elimination at any part. You'll stop losing as much fat.

After this draining process is complete, it's time to re-load your carb reserves by eating carbs normally again for 1-2 days. Loading carbs takes only 1-2 days because the body loves to fill up its carb reserves more quickly than it likes to burn it. Doing this will prevent your metabolism from slowing down, will give you energy, and will make you feel great. Then, once your carb storage areas are full, you can repeat this powerful cycle again, and again, and again. **The days where you slowly drain your carb reserves are referred to as carb-restricted, or low-carb, or easy-on carb days. The days where you re-load your carb reserves are referred to as normal-carb, carb-allowed, or carb-loading days. Let's discuss each of these.**

CARB-RESTRICTED DAYS

Carb-restricted days are designed to slowly and steadily drain your body's carb reserves as well as burn fat. Depending on your activity levels, the draining phase of my Carb Cycle process takes about 2-3 days and is done primarily by reducing your carb intake. In that your body naturally uses your stored carbs and fat deposits to perform everyday activities. Not consuming your normal amount of carbs will deplete your carb reserves. So, as part of my Carb Cycle routine, certain days of the week are designated as carb-restricted days.

What's important to note though, restricting your carbs doesn't mean eliminating them. For now, simply know that carb-restricted days are designed to drain your carb reserves from your body, and that carb-restricted days are *NOT* carb-elimination days. Whenever you cut them completely your body will panic and slow down its metabolism right away! You are supposed to eat carbs every day with every meal, particularly the good, low Glycemic Index carbs like Grains, Green Vegetables, and Fruits.

WHAT CARBS TO RESTRICT

On carb-restricted days all you have to do is cut your carb intake of certain carbs and certain fruits by 50%. What you will cut down on low-carb days are carbs like grains, starches, exotic fruits, and foods that contain processed simple sugars. I'll go over all of your food choices and specifically what carbs exactly you should cut down on low-carb days in the coming chapters. Soon you'll see how easy my program can be.

ANOTHER WAY TO DRAIN CARBS

In discussing the carb drainage process we've only talked about depleting your reserves via restricting your carb consumption. However, you can accelerate the carb drainage process by incorporating exercise into your daily routine. Now, although you don't have to exercise for the Carb Cycle to work, you certainly can and I highly recommend you do.

As a general rule of thumb, if you don't plan on exercising at all, you can cut certain carbs by up to 75% on your low-carb days. I will write more about that later on in this book. However if you do exercise, then on low-carb days you should cut your carbs by no more than 50%. The more you exercise, the more you are going to burn fat and also carbs. Still, unless you exercise 8 hours per day or cut out carbs completely, it will take you 2-3 days to completely deplete your carb storage. Also, you don't want to rush this process and do not have to totally deplete your storage; as long as you are lowering it steadily and slowly for 2-3 days my system works.

CARB-NORMAL DAYS

Once your carb reserves are empty, or close to it, it's time to fill them up again. Doing this is referred to as carb-loading and will happen on your carb-normal days. Loading up carbs takes 1-2 days, less time than burning them off, because whenever you burn carbs you burn a lot of fat simultaneously. Also, the body loves to load carbs whenever its storage is not full. A great feeling you soon will experience when doing your first cycles. Eating on a carb-normal day means you can eat a normal amount of carbs, but they ideally should be the healthy kind of carbs. On carb-normal days it's still important to eat as low glycemic carbs as possible, and avoid eating high glycemic carbs. This will help prevent excess insulin being released too fast and thereby transporting the carbs you eat to your fat cells. Instead, the carbs will be slowly be directed into your natural carb storage areas: the muscles and liver.

Now, that doesn't mean you can't eat some of your favorite carbs on carb-normal days, it's just not a day that encourages blatant disregard for healthy eating. Rather, it's a day to eat and enjoy a normal amount of carbs without worrying about it. Besides, my Carb Cycle Diet allows for a cheat day to eat some less healthy carbs and foods if you "have or like to" on Sundays. More about that shortly.

PUTTING YOUR WEEKLY CARB CYCLE TOGETHER

In combining your carb-normal and carb-restricted (also called low-carb) days, your weekly Carb Cycle should look like this:

DAY	CARB CYCLE RULE
Monday	Carb-*RESTRICTED* (= *50% reduction of all "Basic" Carbs = Grains & Starches along with Exotic Fruits*)
Tuesday	Carb-*RESTRICTED*
Wednesday	Carb-*NORMAL*
Thursday	Carb-*RESTRICTED*
Friday	Carb-*RESTRICTED*
Saturday	Carb-*NORMAL* (*or optionally* **half-day** *RESTRICTED*)
Sunday	Carb-*NORMAL* Sunday is an *optional* day of diet rest – eat anything you like on Sundays, within reason. More about this in upcoming chapters.

As you can see, your Carb Cycle week starts with two back-to-back carb-restricted days. It's important to be strict on these days as your carb reserves are going to be full from eating in a carb-normal manner on part or whole day of Saturday and whole day of Sunday, especially if you used Sunday as a cheat day.

Restricting carbs on **Monday and Tuesday** will probably be easy for most people to do. That's because many people view Monday as the chance to start fresh on their goals. Whether it's work, fitness, or diet, Mondays re-ignite our desire to be better. Use this to your advantage. Decide every Monday to re-commit to my Carb Cycle. The only warning I have is not to go all crazy on Mondays because burning yourself out by depleting your carbs too fast is not going help you. A simple reduction in no more than 50% of all your "basic carbs" (grains and starches) and limiting of "exotic fruits" is all it really takes to get the Carb Cycle started (more about this later!). Rather than trying to push the limits on Monday, set a pace that keeps both your spirit and body going for the whole week!

If you've followed the program properly, by the end of Tuesday your body will be telling you, perhaps screaming, that it's time to eat some more carbs again. Well don't worry, you're not on a constant low-carb or no-carb diet this time, and soon you're going to be able to eat more carbs. Further, knowing that Wednesday is coming soon makes it easier not to cheat on Monday and Tuesday.

Wednesday is a carb-normal day. It's really important to eat carbs normally on this day, as your body needs to replenish its carb storage reserves in order to deplete it again in the coming days. Plus, from a psychological standpoint, Wednesday is a day to truly enjoy eating your carbs. Carbs are "pleasure foods" and your body not only needs them from an energy standpoint, but also from a reward standpoint. With this said though, we're talking about good carbs. This includes things like whole grain breads, certain pastas, oatmeal, high-fiber but sugar-free cereal, fruits, sweet potatoes, brown rice and even some sugar-free, low-fat pancakes or muffins if you'd like, but all in moderation of course.

Thursday and **Friday** are like Monday and Tuesday. They're carb-restricted days and are designed to drain your carb reserves again slowly. After re-filling your carb storage and energy on Wednesday, it's important to be really strict on these days again just as you were on Monday and Tuesday with the exact Carb Cycle Rules. Stay positive and enthusiastic, but don't rush it. Just keep going slowly and steadily. Remember, the weekend is approaching and both weekend days are carb-normal, therefore it's really important and ideal to start the weekend with a low or even empty carb storage system. That way you will be simply re-loading your carb reserves, and if you do cheat, you'll keep any damage to a minimum.

Saturday and Sundays are both carb-normal days. Now you can treat half of Saturday or even the whole day until the evening as a carb-restricted day if you want, that is what I usually do. This is ideal, but it's not critical to your success. However, whenever you do start eating carbs again on Saturday, it's just like you did on Wednesday. Make sure you eat and enjoy carbs normally.

Sunday is a carb-normal day too, but it's also an optional "eat anything you want day." Sunday is "Fun Day". This is your License to Cheat. What this means is that Sunday is the day to enjoy some of the "bad" carbs and foods you tried to stay away from during the week, even on your carb-normal days. Sunday is the day to eat ice cream and pizza, as well as anything else you desire, and it's important to do this for a couple of reasons.

First, there just aren't many people that can be 100% strict with their food intake 100% of the time. We all crave certain foods once in a while, and a few bad meals aren't going to kill your diet. Plus, you've got Monday to re-commit to eating the right way.

Second, after 6 days of eating healthy and two successfully completed weekly carb cycles, you deserve a day off, both physically and mentally. Eating without worrying about anything is like a little positive shock for your system. It reloads your carbs and energy levels and can potentially even give your metabolism a little kick.

Also, because you don't eat that kind of food every day, you are going to enjoy it so much more. Think about it, pizza every day becomes just "normal", but eaten only once per week, can you imagine how good it will taste? And, don't be surprised if you start liking your new, healthy diet so much that you can't wait to go back to the way you eat during the week. That's because a healthy diet will always make you feel totally energetic and great, while a bad diet will eventually make you feel tired and sick. Personally, I usually cheat a little on Sundays, but I don't go to extremes.

I believe that once you get used to healthy eating, you will actually be realizing how bad "unhealthy food" has made you feel. You'll ask yourself, "How in the world did I get by on eating so bad?" The reason is that you probably never realized it before because you didn't know the difference. Personally, after a meal or day of some cheating, I usually can't wait to go back to eating all healthy again.

In any event, my feeling is that if you relax with respect to your food intake once per week, then you're more likely to maintain an overall healthy eating plan for a longer period of time. The same rule applies for holidays. Eat whatever you want on Thanksgiving, Labor Day, or Christmas. Just don't let your Sunday or Holiday eating habits follow you into Monday or too late into Sunday night, that is when you're supposed to get back to the cycle of all healthy food choices. The only Carb Cycle trick and adjustment for holidays is that you can deplete your carb storage for up to three days **before** your "special" holiday-eating day starts. That way, once you start enjoying that particular holiday food you will "first" fill your empty storage which will limit any "damage" to a minimum.

Of course, if you don't feel like eating unhealthy carbs on Sunday or Holidays and prefer all healthy food choices then don't. But whatever you decide, always make sure to eat more carbs on carb-normal days. Otherwise you'll find yourself on a common low-carb diet again that will result in having a constant low or empty carb storage. Doing this will slow down your metabolism and prevent your body from burning as much fat as possible. **Remember, the key to Carb Cycle is not staying constantly full or depleted, but always be in the "Carb Cycle Zone" meaning filling your carb storage for 1-2 days then emptying it slowly over 2-3 days.** So, whatever you do on Sunday, bad or good, make sure you eat and enjoy some carbs.

CARB CYCLE SUMMARY

Eating carbs without feeling guilty and getting fat is welcome news for many people. Particularly for those who are trying to live on a very challenging, permanent low-carb or even no-carb diet. Eating carbs "while" burning lots of fat is even better news – and both is possible with the correct Carb Cycle! Not only do we need to eat carbs but also, most of us want to eat carbs. This is what athletes in great shape do, and what our ancestors also used to do.

So, when it comes to eating carbs, the trick is to cycle them. If you eat too many, you'll get fat. If you eat them normally at all times you'll at best maintain your weight, and if you restrict them permanently, you'll stop burning fat most efficiently. Plus, eating only low-carb in the long-term or completely cutting them out for even just one single meal will probably make you feel miserable and for sure shut-down your metabolism.

That's why my Carb Cycle program works so well. As long as you eat mostly healthy carbs in order to avoid the insulin rollercoaster, and do not ever overfill your carb storage system, you're not going to get fat from eating carbs. Plus, when you *slowly drain* your carb storage areas on the low-carb days *by restricting the right carbs*, you're going to burn fat more effectively and longer than any other diet or program I've ever seen.

With my Carb Cycle Diet you only cycle your basic carbs, which are grains and starches, as well limit exotic fruits. You can keep eating half of your grainy, starchy carbs and full amounts of vegetables, greens, legumes, and northern fruits even on your low-carb days. More about this in the next chapters. Once your carb storage areas are empty, or close to it, you can re-fill them by eating all of your favorite carbs again normally for 1-2 days. Then you can repeat this winning cycle over and over again.

I want you to know that although there are many fine-tuning variations, especially for Advanced Carb Cycle, which we'll discuss in Chapter 9, the basics of my Carb Cycle System are very simple in execution.

It can all be summarized in 3 Key Points:

1) Eat carbs & store them for 1-2 days in your muscles and liver, not your fat cells

2) Reduce (but never cut!) certain specific carbs by 50% and burn your storage off slowly along with any excess fat until your storage is empty or close to it after 2-3 days

3) Repeat this winning Carb Cycle again and again

You'll feel great, never run out of energy, and never have to totally sacrifice carbs – all while getting lean and looking forward to eating all kind of foods on all stages of the Carb Cycle. Through a constant Carb Cycle you will be able to profit from an ongoing metabolic boost, which will create a fat-burning weight-loss cycle after cycle. Plus, unlike other diets or programs, you won't slow down your metabolism and therefore jeopardize future results or sacrifice your energy and well-being.

With that said, the only thing left to decide is: **are you ready to start YOUR FIRST CARB CYCLE?** If so, then let's not waste any more time and immediately begin using your carb storage system the way it was created to be used! In the next chapter I'm going to outline everything you'll need to get going. Welcome to your new, exciting Carb Cycle Lifestyle!

CHAPTER 5

FOOD CHOICES, PORTION SIZES, & MEAL SCHEDULE

Congratulations! You're well on your way to implementing your first Carb Cycle. This chapter is going to be "hands-on," and by that I mean that I'm going to give you a practical guide as to how you can easily begin your very own Carb Cycle Diet. Now, unlike so many other diet books, I'm not going to simply tell you "to eat healthy food or good carbs." Anyone can do that! Instead, I'm going to give you practical tips on how to choose your food wisely along with a detailed schedule as to **WHAT carbs to eat WHEN exactly!** That doesn't mean you'll have to eat exactly the foods or meal combinations I say, it just means that if you need it, I'm providing a detailed eating guide for you. You can always adapt my program to fit your personal lifestyle and individual food choices as long as you cycle the right carbs at the right times in your diet.

Now ideally, like any healthy, common sense diet, my Carb Cycle Diet is based on eating the right quality of lean protein, good carbohydrates, and healthy fats. However, as you know by now, the (R)Evolutionary difference between my diet, and all the others, is the way you arrange and cycle certain carbs you eat. First loading them on Normal-Carb Days, and then depleting them on your Low-Carb Days. This powerful cycle helps you lose weight fast, keeps your metabolism high, and best of all it allows you to still eat carbs regularly with every meal at any point, without ever have to cut carbs out completely for certain meals or even days. No wonder my diet is becoming so popular with so many people.

In this chapter I'm going to introduce you to some basic concepts about food, and how these foods fit into my Carb Cycle Diet. This will include food groups, good choices, portion sizes, when to eat these foods, and some extra tips to maximizing your weight loss results. Then, in the coming chapters, I'll explain the easiest way for starting your Carb Cycle along with an Exercise Routine as well as a 7-Day Quick-Start Meal Example Guide that outlines everything you'll need to get on **_YOUR_** Carb Cycle right away.

FOOD GROUPS:

For now, let's analyze the three basic food types in a little more detail, and discuss good food choices within these categories. I know this might be a review for many of you, but it's really important information. Let's start with protein.

PROTEIN

Protein is an essential part of any diet because it serves as the building blocks for enzymes, antibodies, and hormones. It provides structural material for growth, and helps maintain your muscles, bones, and other tissues. Furthermore, it plays a key role in transporting oxygen, keeping your immune system healthy, and helping in a number of other metabolic processes. Indeed, protein is the foundation of your body and living cells.

When it comes to protein, try to eat natural healthy choices. In general, try to eat more fish and vegetable products, while eating dairy and meat in moderation. Next I've listed some good protein sources.

PROTEIN

CARB CYCLE RULE

► Eat 3-5 Servings every Day

GOOD PROTEIN CHOICES ARE:

- Fish, such as: Salmon, Swordfish, Haddock, Yellow Tail, Halibut, and Tuna
- Egg Whites (or substitutes)
- Lean Poultry such as: Chicken Breast, Turkey Breast, Lean Ground Turkey, Ostrich
- Shrimp, Lobster, and Crab
- Lean Red Meat such as: Top Round Steak, Lean Ground Beef, Top Sirloin Shank, Buffalo, Lean Ham (Note: I suggest you to eat red meat no more than 1-2 times per week, personally I only eat it on special occasions)
- Dairy Products that are non-fat or low-fat and sugar-free such as: Cottage Cheese, Yogurt, Milk, etc.
- Protein Shakes or Meal Replacements, such as Whey or Soy Protein Shakes, Pre-packed Drinks or Bars. NOTE: Make sure to choose low-carb, low-fat, low-sugar and low-calorie products, ideally containing no more than 110-200 Calories per serving and some additional fiber. Count them as a whole snack or meal and do not combine them with other food except an apple or a few nuts.
- Tofu and other Lean Soy Products
- Nuts such as Almonds, Peanuts, etc. also contain Protein
- Beans such as chick peas, black beans, lentils, etc. - which are high in protein *AND* carbohydrates (be aware of this and careful on your low-carb days!)

A balanced, healthy diet should contain some quality protein with every meal or snack you're consuming. As a rule of thumb, your daily protein intake should be about 0.5 grams for each pound of bodyweight. Active people, or athletes, should shoot for even more, up to 1 gram per pound. Now sometimes, it can be hard to find good protein. So, a great way to add some extra protein to your diet is with a protein shake. Simply mix some low-carb whey, or soy protein powder with some water, low-fat soymilk, or non-fat milk. For flavor, you can add some fruit, like blueberries. Then, put in some ice cubes and you've got yourself a delicious, non-fat, low-carb, protein smoothie, that's rich in antioxidants and fiber. If you don't want to mix a shake yourself, there are many good brands that offer pre-packed protein shakes that you can take anywhere you go, and easily store in your car or office. Together with an apple, or a handful of nuts, they make the perfect replacement for a meal or snack.

CARBOHYDRATES

We talked a lot about carbs in chapter three, but as a brief reminder, carbs provide your body and your brain with its main energy as well as many important nutrients. They are naturally stored in your liver and your muscles, and can be cycled in your diet to cause incredible weight loss results. Now, even though my Carb Cycle Diet encourages you to eat carbs at all times, you should still always try to eat as healthy as possible. If you remember, we call these healthy carbs complex carbs, or good carbs. These carbs are loaded with nutrients and have a minimal effect on the release of insulin, thereby further lowering the chances of transforming the carbs you eat into fat.

To simplify and structure your carb choices, we are going to split all good, healthy carbs into 3 groups. These are the types of carbs you should ideally eat and re-arrange in a specific cycle on both your carb-loading and your carb-depleting days. Let me now explain how exactly this is done.

The 3 Carb Cycle Carbohydrate Groups are:

1. **BASIC CARBS = GRAINS & STARCHES**

2. **VEGETABLES & LEGUMES**

3. **FRUITS**

1. BASIC CARBOHYDRATES:

= Grains and Starches

BASIC CARBS

CARB CYCLE RULE

▶ **Eat Normally on Carb-Loading Days**

▶ **Cut by 50% on Low-Carb Days**

GOOD BASIC CARB CHOICES ARE:

- Oatmeal, Barley, Quinoa, etc.
- Brown Rice, Wild Rice, Rice Cakes, etc.
- Potatoes, Sweet Potatoes, Yams, etc.
- Whole Wheat sugar-free Bread and Crackers
- Whole Wheat Pasta
- Beans
- Corn
- Cereal (sugar-free!)
- Any other Grain & Wheat Products

When eating things like bread, pasta, and cereal, always try to eat whole grain varieties. Avoid sugar as much as possible and avoid any processed carbs = foods made from white flour, containing sugar, and/or having too many ingredients. In fact, a good rule to follow is to avoid all white carbs made of "white" sugar and flour. Instead, stick with unsweetened, whole carbs such as brown rice and other whole grain products. If you must indulge in more of the sugary/white carbs, then try to wait until your cheat day.

VEGETABLES & LEGUMES

CARB CYCLE RULE

▶ **Eat 2-4 Servings on all Days,**

Low and Normal-Carb

GOOD VEGETABLE AND LEGUMES CHOICES ARE:

- Broccoli
- Asparagus
- Lettuce
- Onions
- Cucumber
- Zucchini
- Tomatoes
- Spinach
- Mushrooms
- Red/Yellow/Green Peppers
- Cauliflower
- Carrots
- Green Beans & Peas
- Peas
- Artichoke
- Cabbage
- Celery
- Squash & Pumpkin Varieties
- Cabbage
- Salads

You can eat Vegetables and Legumes almost as much as you like, but ideally as part of a regular, balanced program. They will fill you up when you're hungry, and be a good source of fiber, especially on low-carb days.

3. FRUITS:

We are going to split Fruits into 2 Groups:

1) **Northern Fruits**
   = grown in Northern Climates

2) **Exotic or Southern Fruits**
   = grown in Southern Climates

NORTHERN FRUITS

CARB CYCLE RULE

► **Eat 2-4 Servings on all Days,**

Low and Normal-Carb

NORTHERN FRUIT CHOICES ARE:

- Apples
- Pears
- Strawberries
- Blueberries
- Blackberries
- Grapes
- Raspberries
- Plums
- Cherries
- Apricots
- Etc. (other fruits grown in northern climates)

Northern fruit choices tend to contain less sugar and can be eaten for 2-4 servings per day. As I'll reveal shortly, you can eat these foods every day, on both low and normal-carb days.

EXOTIC FRUITS

CARB CYCLE RULE

► **Eat Normally on Carb-Loading Days**

► **Avoid or Eat Sparingly on Low-Carb Days**

EXOTIC FRUIT CHOICES ARE:

- Bananas
- Grapefruits
- Oranges
- Pineapples
- Melons
- Papayas
- Mangos
- Nectarines
- Etc. (other fruits grown in southern climates)

If your goal is to lose weight, these "Exotic Fruits" should ideally only be eaten on your Normal-Carb Days. If you do eat these foods on your low-carb days, then do so sparingly. For example, put only ¼ Banana into your oats or protein shake, instead of a whole one.

FAT

Certain healthy-fats are essential, and if eaten at the right amount can even speed up your metabolism. Small portions of healthy fat, derived from plant sources or fish, should always be part of your daily diet.

When fats are eaten and digested, they become fatty acids. These fatty acids are either saturated, like butter, (usually solid at room temperature,) or, unsaturated, like vegetable oil, (usually liquid at room temperature.) Unsaturated fats have a higher nutritional value and are typically much healthier. On the other hand, saturated fats can lead to all kinds of health problems, especially if eaten too much.

The key when it comes to fat, is to keep it simple. You can do this by limiting most saturated fats, like the type you find in many meats and dairy products. Instead, look for unsaturated fats, like the ones found in vegetable oils, nuts, seeds, and fish. Unsaturated fats are usually also loaded with vitamins. Also, be careful and avoid eating too much in the way of processed fats, such as partially hydrogenated vegetable oils. Although they are still vegetable oils, once they are hydrogenated (artificially hardened), they become much more saturated. There is evidence that those fats, used in many commercially prepared foods, can be harmful, especially in large amounts.

BEWARE OF FAT-FREE

Fat-free foods are a great way to avoid fat, but they're usually loaded with bad carbs. And remember, bad carbs are easily turned into fat. Fat-free is a good way, but only if it is low or no-carb too. Plus, make sure you're not eating something that is overly processed. Fat-free doesn't mean calorie free or healthy.

FAT

CARB CYCLE RULE

▶ **Eat in Moderation on all Days**

GOOD FAT CHOICES ARE:

- Monounsaturated fats found in Nuts and Seeds such as: Almonds, Peanuts, Sunflower Seeds, etc.
- Avocados and Olives
- All natural Vegetable Oils, especially: Olive Oil, Canola Oil, Flax Seed Oil
- Omega-3 Fats found in Fish Oils and Vegetable Oils
- 100% Natural Almond or Peanut Butter

Fat is often "visible", such as in skin on chicken, butter, margarine, solid cooking fats, various oils, salad dressings, and sauces. However, it can also be hidden, like the fat in milk products, processed meats, baked goods, cheese, peanut butter, nuts, seeds, chips, and fried foods. The best way to go is to choose natural, unprocessed foods. Things like nuts, seeds, vegetable oils, and fish oils. Fish oils, and most vegetable oils, such as flax oil are excellent fat sources, as they contain Omega-3 fatty acids, which can help balance cholesterol as well as blood glucose. Avoid processed fat as well as any animal-based fat, which also contains a lot of cholesterol, whenever possible. Also be aware that any over-consumption of fat – even healthy fat – can potentially lead to being overweight. Today, the average American consumes up to 50% of his daily calories from fat, and the rest are mainly carbohydrates. Don't fall into this trap. Aim to eat no more than

20% fat, and make it healthy fat choices. If your Carb Cycle is made of strictly healthy food choices, you can even increase your fat intake a little on your low-carb days. Eat a little bit more fat, like some extra nuts, or try adding an extra tablespoon of olive oil or flax oil to your salad or veggies. However, don't overdo it. Never exceed ½ - 1 handful of nuts, or 1-2 tablespoons of oil. You can also eat a little less fat on your normal-carb days, but generally I would keep your fat consumption moderate and healthy at all times.

FINAL NOTE ON FOOD CHOICES:

All the above listed good Carb Cycle foods should be consumed in their natural, clean form. For example, use plain peanuts, NOT the salted ones, which have extra salt, sugar, and other additives. Avoid any processed or refined foods that are low in nutrients but high in sugar, fat, or salt. These include processed breads, cereals, creamy sauces, oily or buttery foods, etc.. Grill or steam your food whenever possible. Avoid butter, baked or deep-fried food, and don't forget to watch any liquids you consume, especially sodas, smoothies, shakes, and fruit juices. Also be aware of calorie-loaded additives like gravy, salad dressings, and fatty or sugary spices. Read labels and ask questions. If there are too many ingredients, be careful. Remember that your body thinks in terms of nutrients, and not in calories. The more "one ingredient" foods you choose, the better.

On the next page is a quick chart you can reference as to the food categories and how you ideally re-arrange them on both Normal-Carb days, as well as Low-Carb days.

CARB CYCLE FOOD RULES

CATEGORY	NORMAL-CARB DAY	LOW-CARB DAY
Protein	3-5 Servings Per Day	3-5 Servings Per Day
Carbohydrates – *Basic* *= Grains & Starches*	**Eat Normal**	**Cut by 50%**
Carbohydrates – *Vegetables & Legumes*	2-4 Servings Per Day	2-4 Servings Per Day
Carbohydrates – *Northern Fruits*	2-4 Servings Per Day	2-4 Servings Per Day
Carbohydrates – *Exotic Fruits*	**Eat Normal**	**Avoid or eat sparingly**
Fat	In Moderation	In Moderation

WHEN TO EAT

When you eat depends mostly on your personal routine. However, I recommend that once you get up, you should eat breakfast within about 30 minutes, and then eat every 2-3 hours after that. If you're planning on exercising first thing in the morning, then eat breakfast right after doing this. Also, remember to drink 1-2 glasses of water as soon as you wake up. Your best choice is to follow a Daily Meal Schedule like this:

DAILY MEAL SCHEDULE:

1. **BREAKFAST**

2. **MID-MORNING SNACK**

3. **LUNCH**

4. **MID-AFTERNOON SNACK**

5. **DINNER**

6. **OPTIONAL: GOOD NIGHT SNACK**

On the next two pages, let's go over this schedule for a moment and examine what each meal should consist of.

*Note: To make sure there are no misunderstandings, I included the Basic Carb Cycle Rules in the following breakdown marked with a " * ".*

1. BREAKFAST:

- ▶ 1 Portion of Protein
- ▶ 1 Portion of **Basic Carbs***
- ▶ 1 Portion of **Fruits*** or Vegetables
- ▶ 1 Portion Healthy Fat, especially on low-carb days
- ▶ 1-2 Glasses of Water
- ▶ Optional: Coffee or Tea
- ▶ Suggested: 1 Multivitamin Supplement

CARB CYCLE RULE FOR BREAKFAST:
½ Basic Carbs & No Exotic Fruits**
on Low-Carb Days (Mon/Tue, Thur/Fri)

2. MID-MORNING SNACK:

- ▶ 1 Portion of Protein/Healthy Fat/**Fruit*** Mix
  or Healthy Carb Snack*
- ▶ 1-2 Glasses of Water or Tea

CARB CYCLE RULE FOR AM SNACK:
No Exotic Fruits or Healthy Carb Snack**
on Low-Carb Days (Mon/Tue, Thur/Fri)

3. LUNCH:

- ▶ 1 Portion of Protein
- ▶ 1 Portion of **Basic Carbs***
- ▶ 1 Portion of Vegetables and/or Legumes
- ▶ 1 Portion of Healthy Fat
- ▶ 1-2 Glasses of Water or Tea

CARB CYCLE RULE FOR LUNCH:
½ Basic Carbs on Low-Carb Days (Mon/Tue, Thur/Fri)*

4. MID-AFTERNOON SNACK:

- ▶ 1 Portion of Protein/Healthy Fat/**Fruit*** Mix **or Healthy Carb Snack***
- ▶ 1-2 Glasses of Water or Tea
- ▶ Optional: Coffee or Tea

CARB CYCLE RULE FOR PM SNACK:
No Exotic Fruits or Healthy Carb Snack*
on Low-Carb Days (Mon/Tue, Thur/Fri)*

5. DINNER:

- ▶ 1 Portion of Protein
- ▶ 1 Portion of Basic **Carbs***
- ▶ 1-2 Portions of Vegetables and Salad
- ▶ 1 Portion of Healthy Fat
- ▶ 1-2 Glasses of Water or Tea

CARB CYCLE RULE FOR DINNER:
½ or No Basic Carbs on Low-Carb Days
(Mon/Tue, Thur/Fri)*

6. OPTIONAL NIGHT SNACK:

- ▶ ½ - 1 Portion of Protein
- ▶ Optional: some small amount of low-sugar / high-fiber **Carbs*** or healthy Fat like some Peanuts or Almonds or some cut Apple or Pear slices
- ▶ Good Night Tea

CARB CYCLE RULE FOR NIGHT SNACK:
No Exotic Fruits on Low-Carb Days (Mon/Tue, Thur/Fri)*

Note: *Coffees and Teas always sugar-free, especially on low-carb days and if then with Non- or Low-Fat Milk or Soymilk*

PORTION SIZES

As we get into the next chapter, we're going over some exact Meals Plans and recommendations for implementing my Carb Cycle Diet. To do this most effectively, I don't want you to have to count calories or grams. That's too much work and something you just can't do long term. Instead, I want you to get used to eating food in terms of Portion Sizes. Knowing what a Portion Size is will help you more easily make decisions and prevent you from having to worry too much about how much you're eating. And isn't that the point of adopting a better way of eating? Never having to worry about calories and grams or obsessing over the food you eat.

PROTEIN PORTION:

One Portion is about the Size of your Palm (without the Fingers)

For Protein Powder, which is denser, usually 1 Scoop is enough

If you eat Fish, a Portion Size can be a little bigger = 1-2 times your Palm Size.

CARBOHYDRATES PORTION:

1) BASIC CARBS
GRAINS & STARCHES:

One portion is about 1 times
your palm size (without fingers)

2) VEGETABLES & LEGUMES:

One portion is about 1-2 handfuls

3) FRUITS:

One portion is about ½ to 1 of your palm size,
depending how watery the fruit is. The more water
it contains, the bigger a portion can be.

FAT PORTION:

One portion of Nuts and Seeds:
A small Handful

One Portion of Oils:
1-2 Tablespoons

One Portion of Almond or Peanut Butter:
1-2 Teaspoons

EXTRA NOTE ON FAT PORTIONS:
Healthy Fat is added in moderation to 2-4 meals, ideally used as an additive (like some nuts into oatmeal), or for cooking or dressings (like a tablespoon to cook meat with or fix a salad).

Fat-Exception 1: If you use nuts or seeds as a whole meal or snack, which is especially beneficial on your low-carb days, go for a whole handful of it, in order to get some more protein. Be aware that almost every food contains some fat. Don't worry too much that you're not getting enough fat, especially if you still want to lose weight. Just make sure to add some small amounts of healthy fat choices to 2-3 meals and you will be fine.

Fat-Exception 2: On low-carb days, you can and should allow yourself to eat a little more healthy fats or at least make sure not to skip them, especially when you get too hungry. However, incorporate only good fats such as Olive Oil, Omega-3 Supplements, Avocados, or all-natural nuts and seeds like Almonds.

If you do eat a handful of nuts as a snack make sure you don't eat the whole bag. Fat calories can quickly add up. Some additional small amounts of healthy fat on your low-carb days can actually give you some extra energy as well as speed up your fat burning metabolism, tricking your body to think that there is no need to hold on to it since you are still eating it in small but frequent amounts.

THE 7 PM EVENING RULE

Besides making sure you eat breakfast every day and eat a meal or snack at least every 3 hours, your meals should ideally get a little smaller towards the evening hours. Cutting down on your basic carbs at night is a very simple but effective guideline that I personally always follow and encourage you to do as well. Concentrate on eating most of your carbs earlier in the day. This is the time that you typically need more energy anyway. At night, stick more to protein, vegetables, and greens. If you are still hungry at night, try an herbal tea with some sweetener, an apple, or some nuts like almonds, but only in moderation. For anybody who is used to eating most of their daily food at night, and/or skips breakfast, it's important to break that cycle as quickly as possible. The good news is that as soon as you start eating breakfast and regular snacks and meals during daytime, after a few days it will be easy not to overeat anymore at night time. One of the benefits will be a more healthy sleep because your body will not be busy digesting huge amounts of food but can focus on recuperating and balancing your hormone- as well as nervous system. Many experts believe growth hormone is released more efficiently when going to bed without eating too much food the last hours before. Based on my experience, this is true and another reason to eat less at night. Without side-tracking too much, growth hormone is integral in building muscle, repairing tissue, and burning fat.

TIP: I usually suggest when first starting your Carb Cycle Meal Schedule to set your alarm on your phone for every 2-3 hours so you won't miss any meals or snacks.

CONCLUSION

Now that we've discussed what the 3 main elements of food are, the good choices within each category, and the Carb Cycle rules associated with these – it's time to outline and choose your individually customized Carb Cycle Schedule and Meal Plan. So, in the next 2 Chapters that's exactly what we'll do.

CHAPTER 6

IMPLEMENTING YOUR OWN CARB CYCLE

HOW TO IMPLEMENT CARB CYCLE INTO YOUR OWN DIET

There are two simple ways to implement the Carb Cycle into your diet:

OPTION 1: You can follow my Carb Cycle Diet and all of the Carb Cycle Rules as much as possible in regards to the food choices, portion sizes, and times you eat. There is no need to be too meticulous and start counting calories, grams, or carbs, but I will discuss this a little more in the next couple of chapters. To get in great shape it just isn't necessary to count calories, or measure the grams of the foods and carbs you eat. I personally never do this but simply go by the portion rules, food choices, and other simple Guidelines I'm explaining in this book.

OPTION 2: If for whatever reason you don't want to follow the exact above option, you can still implement my Carb Cycle System with your current eating habits, food choices, or any other diet or food program you're already on. All you have to do is cut your basic carbs (= grains and starches) in half on your low-carb days along with limiting exotic fruits, and then eat them in your usual manner on your normal-carb days. If you follow a diet that is based on allergies or special medical food requirements then consult with your doctor beforehand. Now, I do not encourage you to start cycling your current diet, especially if it's based on unhealthy food choices. It's better to put an effort into making your food choices as healthy as possible and splitting up your meals accordingly by following the "Eat Breakfast, then every 3 Hours" Rule. That way you will get the fastest and healthiest results possible. However, my Carb Cycle Diet is so powerful that you will get results in any event.

FIT IN 3 STAGES FOR EVERYBODY

Over the years I put together three Carb Cycle Stages you can and should choose from based on your current Fitness and Experience Level. For any starter or anybody who was "off" eating healthy and exercising I strongly advise you start with STAGE 1. Now let me briefly explain the three Stages. They will put you on the perfect path to your own Carb Cycle, whatever fitness level you are on at this point:

THE 3 CARB CYCLE STAGES

Each one of the three Carb Cycle Stages is 30 days long: Stage 1 is for starting the Carb Cycle afresh after time off or for the first time ever. Stage 2 is for intermediate fitness levels. Stages 1 and 2 are all you really need to achieve a fit, lean, and healthy body. However, if you want to go further for that extra lean and chiseled body, then there's Stage 3, Advanced Carb Cycle. For anybody new to a fit and healthy lifestyle, it's important and most efficient to start with Stage 1 and 2 at the beginning. Further, there is a "Stage 4" which will allow you to maintain your achieved success. More about this in Chapter 10 - Carb Cycle for Life.

Online, there will be a sign-up option for a day-by-day three month plan you can join - starting with Day One of Stage 1 all the way up to Day 90 of Stage 3, followed by Stage 4 to maintain your weight loss results.

Sign-up to the Carb Cycle Newsletter or Twitter to stay tuned at: WWW.CARBCYCLE.COM or WWW.TWITTER.COM/CARBCYCLE

STAGE 1

STARTER CARB CYCLE
FOR FIRST 30 DAYS

▶ *START CARB CYCLE WITH YOUR NORMAL*
FOODS AND ADD MORE HEALTHY CHOICES

▶ *EXERCISE LEVEL 1:*
WORKOUT FOR 15-30 MINUTES DAILY

CARB CYCLE: Start by cutting all Basic Carbs in half on Mon/Tue/Thur/Fri/Sat and eat them normally on Wed/Sat-Eve/Sun. Start paying more attention to what food choices you eat and switch to more healthy choices while doing your first couple of Carb Cycles.

EXERCISE: Start walking every day for 15 minutes and do a simple 7 minute toning & stretching workout 2-4 times per week. Another option is to workout 7-10 minutes in the morning, and 7-10 minutes in the afternoon or evening. Optionally, for an extra fat-burn kick: 2-3 times per week, add a 7-15 Minute Walk first thing in the morning, right after getting up. Drink water before and eat breakfast right after.

Note: *In Chapter 8 - "How to Exercise with Carb Cycle" - we'll talk more about Physical Activity and these 3 Exercise Levels!*

STAGE 2

INTERMEDIATE CARB CYCLE
FOR SECOND 30 DAYS

▶ *CARB CYCLE YOUR FOODS AND CHANGE*
TO MOSTLY HEALTHY CHOICES

▶ *EXERCISE LEVEL 2:*
WORKOUT FOR 30-60 MINUTES DAILY

CARB CYCLE: Keep your Carb Cycle by cutting basic carbs 50% on your low-carb days while switching to mostly healthy food choices, especially from Monday to Saturday.

EXERCISE: Do a cardio session - such as walking, biking, hiking, elliptical, etc. - 1 time daily for 30 minutes or 2 times daily for 15 minutes. Add a 15-30 minute toning workout 3-5 times per week, ideally on Mon/Tue/Thur/Fri to further empty your carb storage on your low-carb days. Stretch out a little before, between, and after your workouts. For an extra metabolism & fat-burn kick: try to add 15 Min of empty stomach cardio time first thing in the morning 3-5 times per week. Keep this Stage for 30 days or as long as you like, then either switch to Stage 3, Advanced Carb Cycle, in order to maximize your program and chisel down even more, or go directly to Stage 4, Carb Cycle for Life, which is explained in Chapter 10.

STAGE 3

ADVANCED CARB CYCLE
OPTIONAL AFTER STAGE 1 & 2

▶ *TEMPORARILY MAXIMIZE*
YOUR CARB CYCLE BY CUTTING CARBS
UP TO 75% ON LOW-CARB DAYS

▶ *EXERCISE LEVEL 3:*
WORKOUT 60 MINUTES OR MORE DAILY

CARB CYCLE: Cut down your basic carbs from 50% to 75% on low-carb days. Never go below 50-75 grams/day and never skip Normal-Carb Days to refill your storage accordingly! Change to only healthy food choices, especially from Mon-Sat. Cut cheating with processed, sugary, and fatty foods or limit to a minimum. Instead load-up with mostly healthy foods such as fruits and other natural, healthy choices on the weekends.

EXERCISE: Ideally split up your workouts in 2-3 daily segments. For example do a 15-30 min empty stomach morning workout, another 15 min one midday, and another 15-30 one in the evening. Do cardio for at least 30-45 minutes every day, mostly at a medium intensity pace except 2-3 times per week at a higher pace. Toning or weight workouts should be done every day for 15-30 min or every other day for 30-60 min. After toning up with Stage 1 and Stage 2 - this Stage can get you in absolute Bikini Shape whenever you are ready for it by using Stage 1 and 2 firsthand. **NEVER GO TO THIS STAGE IF YOU ARE A STARTER OR RE-STARTING!** Remember, to lose fat and achieve top shape is a journey, not a sprint, in order to maintain it for a lifetime & keep results steady.

CARB CYCLE IN EMERGENCY OR STRESSFUL SITUATIONS

I know from my own experience that on some days it's very easy to follow a healthy diet, but on other days it can be extremely difficult. Life happens. The most important tip I can give you in order to avoid any last minute emergencies, or excuses to not eating healthy, is to always go over your next day's meal plan and foods the evening before. Here you can make some basic notes and preparations for what you'll be eating.

Also, it helps to print and keep your Basic Meal Schedule in your wallet, especially in the beginning weeks. Doing this will remind you whether it is a low-carb or normal-carb day as well as when and what to eat. Whenever you know that you are going to be very busy, either prepare your meals in advance and bring them with you, or know and decide in advance where you can go get them during the day. That way, when it's time to eat or snack, you'll never eat a bad meal or skip a meal.

It helps to make a plan of what exactly you eat the night before as well as print and keep your Daily Meal Schedule in your wallet.

Personally, I always keep some salt-free nuts like almonds or peanuts in my car, as well as 2-4 low-calorie, low-carb protein/meal replacement shakes for emergencies. Plus, I usually bring 1-2 Apples with me and make sure I have plenty of water or tea with me to go for hours. Whenever you get super busy, have unexpected marathon meetings, or "must attend" lunches, or whatever else, you can eat your nuts & apples and drink your protein along with never running out of water. It's worth putting that little extra effort in every night and think ahead. Whenever you are ordering out make sure to choose as healthy as possible. The good thing is that most restaurants offer healthy choices and accommodate for people eating carb-conscious. Don't hesitate to be clear and a little assertive in these situations.

If you're ever in a situation where you just can't avoid eating poorly, because someone either cooked for you, or there is no way to avoid the foods being served, just enjoy what you eat and keep the amount as little as possible. Do not feel bad after! Being on a constant Carb Cycle and getting right back on whenever you fall off will make sure that there will be as little or no long-term damage.

If you fall off your bike or horse – don't stay down feeling bad – just jump back on and keep riding. It's the Cycle of Life – your life - and now you are officially on it. **WELCOME TO YOUR CARB CYCLE!**

CARB CYCLE MEAL PLAN RULES:

- **What day and how to start:** Ideally you should start your Carb Cycle on a Monday but you can start it on any other day too. In case you were on a constant low-carb diet, remember that it's important to eat carbs every few days. You can only drain your natural carb storage areas if they're filled up on a regular basis. And the draining process is where most of the fat loss occurs. So, it's a good idea to eat a little more carbs the day before you start your first carb cycle. Therefore, practically, your best point to start your first Carb Cycle is either Wednesday or Sunday by eating some "more" carbs on either day, then start your first low-carb day the following day which is Monday or Thursday. **Yes, I just told you to start your diet by eating *MORE* carbs. Not a bad way to start a new diet - isn't it!**

- **Eat smaller but more often:** Eat 5-6 smaller meals per day instead of 2-3 large ones, including snacks. Keeping your meals more frequent and smaller makes them digest more efficiently and speeds up your metabolism. Further, eating smaller but more frequently during daytime hours will shrink your stomach and make you less hungry after 7 pm, when you should actually eat less; especially carbs.

- **Weekly Carb Cycle Summary:** Once again, the Carb Cycle works like this: Cut your Basic Carbohydrates = Grains and Starches in half along with limiting Exotic Fruits on Monday and Tuesday, Thursday and Friday, and optionally half of Saturday. Eat frequent protein, vegetables and greens, as well as 1-2 apples or pears any day of the week. Remember that low-carb doesn't mean "no-carb." *NEVER* go "no-carb" but stick to the 50%, or in case you later on like to try an Advanced Carb Cycle, maximally 75% Rule. Less is not better in this case and some carbs belong in every single meal of your diet. Do not try to adjust the days of this weekly Cycle and in case you fall off just get back on it without trying to balancing it out. For example, if you eat more carbs on Tuesday by accident or whatever reason, don't make Wed a low-carb day. Otherwise, you will be adjusting it back and forth and just be on another low-carb diet with a lot of messed-up meals and days.

- **You *MUST* load carbs always:** Make sure to remember that you must eat normal carb amounts on at least Wednesday and Sunday! You need to eat carbs on these days in order to replenish your carb storage, give yourself energy, and prevent your metabolism from slowing down. If you want to push your weight loss results, increase the cycle intensity a little and make Saturday an optional low-carb day as well. However, Wednesday and Sunday you *NEED* to eat more carbs! Otherwise you are just on a constant low-carb diet again and this is not what we want!

- **The healthier & natural the better:** Ideally, remove all processed foods from your diet during your low-carb days. Remember, processed foods are usually mixed with lots of sugar, fat, salt, and other unhealthy, high-calorie ingredients that potentially slow down or even destroy your diet. Examples are fatty pizza & pasta dishes, fried foods, sodas, cake, cookies, breads, bagels, and muffins. Replace them with all-natural, nourishing foods like the ones I've listed in this book. Choose more "one ingredient foods" which are 100% natural foods. For example, an apple has only one ingredient listed in its ingredient list: apple. If you are a starter - use the three stages I talked about earlier in order to slowly adjust your body to more healthy food choices.

- **License to Cheat:** On the first few days of your diet try to stay away from any bad food as much as possible to maximize your success & totally clean out your body. Then, if you'd like to, start adding some not-so-healthy food choices as cheating meals 1-2 times per week again. Preferably on Sundays, but only if you like and/or have to. Another variation is that you may not want to use Sunday as your cheat day. Saturdays might be a better day for you to relax with respect to your food. Also, if it fits your work or lifestyle better, you don't have to start your Carb Cycle on Monday, but can start any day you'd like. Just keep the cycle of going 2-3 days low-carb, followed by 1-2 days of normal carbs. Whatever you do, make sure to keep the basic protein, carbohydrate, and fat ratios I wrote about and to cycle your carbs accordingly. Use your license to cheat wisely!

- **Watch what you drink:** Drink only water or other non-caloric drinks. Avoid any sodas, even if calorie-free, or at least limit them to an absolute minimum. If you consume 100% natural fruit juices, count them as a whole meal and try to put them into your normal-carb days. Put an effort into drinking at least 8-12 glasses of water per day, especially in the morning and afternoon hours. This will help keep your metabolism running high and burning fat like crazy. In fact, dehydration is one of the worst enemies of a healthy, fat-burning metabolism, so make sure to stay well hydrated all day long. If you compare your metabolism to a burning fire, water is to your metabolism what oxygen is to a fire.

- **A trick for holidays and parties**: There is one special rule to change the days of your low and normal-carb days: Holidays or exceptional Festivities such as Birthdays or other Occasions. For example, every Thanksgiving, which falls on a Thursday, I go low-carb for Mon, Tue, *AND* Wed (usually a normal-carb day) and then load carbs on the "special occasion" in this case Thanksgiving on Thursday (usually a low-carb day). Then, on Fri & Sat I go low-carb again, Sunday back to normal-carb and the regular cycle. This way I make sure to go into any special eating "reason" with an empty carb storage which will keep any damage to an absolute minimum. Use this trick and adjustment rarely and do not abuse it as an excuse to eat bad too often and go back to your normal carb cycle days as soon as possible afterwards.

CHAPTER 7

7-DAY QUICK START
MEAL EXAMPLES

CHOOSING FROM A VARIETY OF MEAL COMBINATIONS

The great thing about implementing your Carb Cycle Meal Plan is that there are probably thousands of individual, creative ways to prepare your daily meals. After all my years on the Carb cycle I still discover new meal combinations all the time. You can find healthy low-carb or normal-carb recipes just about everywhere at bookstores and on the internet. For this reason, I didn't want this book to be another recipe loaded book. Wherever you find your recipes or in whatever way you combine your foods, what matters is that you Cycle the right Carbs accordingly.

When it comes to your individual meals and snacks, don't hesitate to switch and substitute other food choices as long as they're in the same food groups you've learned about. For example, you can start your day with some oats and an egg white omelet. If you don't want the omelet, try a protein shake, salmon, cottage cheese, or any of the other good protein choices. The same rule applies for the oatmeal. You can substitute it with barley, potatoes, a high fiber/sugar-free cereal, and so on. Over time you will find your own preferences, and will probably begin to eat the same types of meals every day. Finding and keeping your own individual routine that stays similar or even the same every day is always the best thing to do when it comes to eating as healthy as possible.

IF YOU STILL NEED SOME VARIETY, YOU CAN KEEP CHANGING THE COMBINATION OF YOUR MEALS

The following 7-Day Morning to Evening Meal Plan Examples outlay a Variety of Meal Options which will allow you to quick-start your Carb Cycle Diet and guide you through your first weeks of your Carb Cycle. It will instantly jump start your metabolism and make your body burn fat. Best of all, you can continue this winning cycle for as long as you want. Keep in mind, the simpler you keep your meals, the easier your entire plan will be to follow.

As a reminder and as mentioned in previous chapters, you should be eating some healthy protein, healthy fat in moderation, as well as vegetables and greens multiple times per day. You can also eat non-exotic fruits whenever you want. On the other hand, make sure to cut "Basic Carbs" like Grains and Starches accordingly by 50% along with eliminating Exotic Fruits on your low-carb days, and then eat full portions of all carbs again on your normal-carb days. Also, especially on those low-carb days, you should try to eliminate all simple "bad" carbs, also called sugar-carbs, as much as possible. If you want or must eat these "bad carbs," save them for your cheat day, or at the very least, eat them only on your normal-carb days, when you actually are re-filling your carb storage system.

A wonderful side effect of being on a constant conscious Carb Cycle is that you'll be less likely to crave sugary and fatty foods and drinks soon. Your body will soon start to enjoy your new healthy choices, along with having its carb storage first filled and then depleted in an ongoing and slow cycle. Once you experience the feeling of being on a carb cycle for yourself, you'll never want to go back to your old way of eating.

Let me now give you a whole week of Monday to Sunday Carb Cycle Meal and Snack Examples from morning to evening.

A WHOLE WEEK OF MEAL EXAMPLES

MONDAY EXAMPLE
= *LOW-CARB DAY**

BREAKFAST:
▶ *Egg White Omelet (3-5 Egg Whites) with ¼ Avocado*
▶ **HALF PORTION* of Oatmeal,** *mixed with 1 Tablespoon of Almonds, and either 1 Tablespoon of Blueberries* **OR** *1/2 of an apple cut in small pieces*
▶ *1-2 Glasses of Water*
▶ *Optional: Coffee or Tea*
▶ *1 Multivitamin Supplement*

MID-MORNING SNACK:
▶ *1 Apple or Pear with a handful of Almonds or Peanuts* **OR** *1 Low-Carb Protein Shake*
▶ *1-2 Glasses of Water or Tea*

LUNCH:
▶ **HALF PORTION*** *of Steamed Wild Rice*
▶ *1 Portion of White Turkey*
▶ *1 Portion of Steamed Broccoli*
▶ *1 Small Salad with Balsamic Vinegar & 1-2 Tablespoon of Olive Oil*
▶ *1-2 Glasses of Water or Unsweetened Iced Tea*

MID-AFTERNOON SNACK:

- *1 Low-Carb Protein Shake **OR** a handful of Nuts*
- *1-2 Glasses of Water*
- *Optional: Coffee or Tea*

DINNER:

- *1 Portion of Grilled Ahi Tuna or Salmon*
- *Steamed Vegetables with 1-2 Tablespoon of Olive Oil, or 1/2 Avocado.*
- *Optional: **HALF PORTION* of Baked Potato***
- *1-2 Glasses of Water or Tea*

OPTIONAL NIGHT-SNACK:

- *1 Low-Carb Yogurt & ½ Apple*
- *1 Herbal Tea (beware of caffeine if you're sensitive!)*

NOTE: *Every day drink AT LEAST 8-12 GLASSES OF WATER. Optionally, drink 1-2 green teas and/or 1-3 Coffee's, both sugar & fat-free, especially on low-carb days.*

TUESDAY EXAMPLE
= *LOW-CARB DAY**

BREAKFAST:
- *1 Protein Shake: 1 Scoop of Low-Carb Protein Powder mixed with Water or some Nonfat Milk or low-fat Soymilk. Add some Blueberries (or any Berries) OR* **1/2 Banana***
- *OPTIONAL: Add some Ice Cubes and some Peppermint Oil drops. For extra Fiber add* **Oatmeal (HALF PORTION*)**

OR Breakfast Example 2:
- *A Low-Carb Protein Boost Frittata with 3-5 Egg Whites, Cut Lox, Arugula, Olive Oil*
- **1-2 Rye Crackers*** *with 1 Tablespoon of Hummus*

Either Breakfast with:
- *1-2 Glasses of Water*
- *Optional: Coffee or Tea*
- *1 Multivitamin Supplement*

MID-MORNING SNACK:
- *1 Apple or Pear with a handful of Almonds or Peanuts* **OR,** *1 Low-Carb Protein Shake*
- *1-2 Glasses of Water or Tea*

LUNCH:
- *1 Portion Lean Grilled Chicken Breast*
- *1 Portion Steamed Vegetables,*
- **HALF PORTION of Sweet Potato OR** *Butternut Squash (no added fat or sugar) with 1 Tablespoon of Olive Oil*
- *1-2 Glasses of Water or Unsweetened Iced Tea*

MID-AFTERNOON SNACK:

▶ *1 Protein Rich Low-Carb Yogurt **OR,** Low-Carb Protein Shake with Handful of Peanuts*

▶ *1-2 Glasses of Water*

▶ *Optional: Coffee or Tea*

DINNER:

▶ *1 Portion Vegetable Soup Mix with Fish or Tofu*

▶ *Salad with natural Spices & Balsamic Vinaigrette & either Olive Oil OR 1/2 Avocado*

▶ *OPTIONAL: **HALF PORTION* of Wheat Toast OR,** 1 **Whole Grain Cracker***

▶ *1-2 Glasses of Water or Tea*

OPTIONAL NIGHT-SNACK:

▶ *Handful of Almonds and/or 1 Low-Carb Yogurt*

▶ *1 Herbal Tea*

WEDNESDAY EXAMPLE
= _NORMAL-CARB DAY*_

BREAKFAST:
▶ _Egg White Omelet (3-5 Egg Whites) with Mushrooms, Peppers, and Tomatoes_
▶ **FULL PORTION* of Oatmeal OR, Sugar-Free Cereal,** _mixed with Choice of 1 Fruit (**Exotic*** or Normal)_
▶ _1-2 Glasses of Water_
▶ _Optional: Coffee or Tea_
▶ _1 Multivitamin Supplement_

MID-MORNING SNACK:
▶ **_1 Banana* or Orange* OR, 1-2 Brown Rice Cakes*_** _with 1-2 Tablespoons of non-fat Cottage Cheese and Sprinkled Pepper_
▶ _1-2 Glasses of Water or Tea_

LUNCH:
▶ _1 Portion Grilled Swordfish or Chicken Breast_
▶ _1 Portion of Steamed Vegetables_
▶ _1 **FULL Portion of Brown Rice* or Wild Rice**._
▶ _OPTIONAL DESSERT- **Bowl of any Fruit***_
▶ _1-2 Glasses of Water or Unsweetened Iced Tea_

MID-AFTERNOON SNACK:

▶ *1 Low-Fat/Low-Sugar Muffin* OR, 1 handful of Dried Dates* or Prunes OR, a Sugar-free Fruit Juice**

▶ *1-2 Glasses of Water*

▶ *Optional: Coffee or Tea*

DINNER:

▶ *1 Whole Wheat Burrito*: Add 1 portion of grilled chicken or turkey with 1-2 Tablespoons of healthy salsa. OPTIONAL: add some non-fat cheese, non-fat sour cream, and some black beans. Roll, serve & enjoy. OPTIONAL: **some cut exotic fruits*** as a dessert (it's a normal-carb day – enjoy!)*

OR, DINNER EXAMPLE 2:

▶ *1 Portion of Baked Salmon with **FULL Portion of Whole Wheat Angel Hair Pasta*** on a bed of Arugula Salad. Add Lemon Juice, Olive Oil, Capers & Garlic Dressing (Note: this is one of my favorite Normal-Carb Dishes)*

With either Dinner:

▶ *1-2 Glasses of Water or Tea*

OPTIONAL NIGHT-SNACK:

▶ *Handful of Sliced Melon* Pieces OR, other Fruit Choice*

▶ *Herbal Tea*

THURSDAY EXAMPLE
= *LOW-CARB DAY**

BREAKFAST:
- 1 Portion of Smoked Salmon (Lox) with 1 Portion of Salad and Tomatoes, 1-2 tbsp. of Olive Oil
- **1 Sugar-free Whole Wheat Cracker* OR, HALF of a piece of Wheat Toast***
- 1 Glass of Water
- Optional: Coffee or Tea
- 1 Multivitamin Supplement

MID-MORNING SNACK:
- 1 Apple with a handful of Almonds OR, 1 Low-Carb Protein Shake
- 1-2 Glasses of Water or Tea

LUNCH:
- 1 Portion of Extra-Lean Chicken or Soy Burger on **HALF of a Whole Wheat Bun*** (= half the Bread only!), add Salad with Peppers, Onions, Tomatoes. Some Balsamic Vinaigrette & 1-2 Tablespoons of Olive Oil
- 1-2 Glasses of Water or Iced Tea

MID-AFTERNOON SNACK:

▶ *1 Low-Carb Protein Shake **OR,** Apple or Pear with 1 Handful of Almonds or Peanuts*
▶ *1-2 Glasses of Water*
▶ *Optional: Coffee or Tea*

DINNER:

▶ *1 Portion Grilled or Poached Salmon Steak*
▶ *1 Portion of Steamed Spinach with Freshly Squeezed Lemon Juice*
▶ ***HALF PORTION** of dry Sweet Potato**
▶ *Put some Olive Oil over Sweet Potato*
▶ *1-2 Glasses of Water or Tea*

OPTIONAL NIGHT-SNACK:

▶ *Handful of Seasonal Non-Exotic Fruits like Grapes or Cherries, **OR,** a Low-Carb Yogurt*
▶ *Herbal Tea*

FRIDAY EXAMPLE
= _LOW-CARB DAY*_

BREAKFAST:
- *A bowl of non-fat Cottage Cheese mixed with * with a handful of Berries*
- **1 Rye Cracker* with 1 Teaspoon of Honey***

OR, BREAKFAST EXAMPLE 2:
- **HALF PORTION of Oatmeal*** *mixed with Low-Carb Protein Powder. Add Flaxseeds or liquid Flax-Oil, and a handful of Blueberries. Mix with Water or fat-free Milk or low-fat Soymilk*

Either Breakfast with:
- *1-2 Glasses of Water*
- *1 Multivitamin Supplement*
- *Optional: Coffee or Tea*

MID-MORNING SNACK:
- *1 Apple and a handful of Almonds or Peanuts* **OR,** *1 Low-Carb Protein Shake*
- *1-2 Glasses of Water or Tea*

LUNCH:
- *A Large Green Salad with canned oil-free Tuna, ½ Avocado, Red/Green/Yellow Peppers, Olive Oil & Balsamic Vinegar*
- *OPTIONAL: Add some fat-free Cheese for a tasty Protein Boost.*
- **HALF PORTION of Whole Wheat Bread* OR, 1 Whole Grain Cracker***
- *1-2 Glasses of Water or unsweetened Iced Tea*

MID-AFTERNOON SNACK:

- *1 Brown Rice Cake* with Turkey Breast & Pepper Hummus OR, 1 Low-Carb Protein Shake with a Handful of Peanuts*
- *1-2 Glasses of Water*
- *Optional: Coffee or Tea*

DINNER:

- *Tofu-Vegetable Bowl: 1 Potion of Tofu mixed with cut Asparagus, Carrots, Red Bell Pepper, and Sweet Peas. Cook together. OPTIONAL: add HALF PORTION of Brown Rice* or Wild Rice*
- *1-2 Glasses of Water or Tea*

OPTIONAL NIGHT-SNACK:

- *1 Apple or Pear*
- *Low-Carb Yogurt OR, Handful of Nuts*
- *Herbal Tea*

SATURDAY EXAMPLE
= *NORMAL-CARB DAY**
OR,
OPTIONAL HALF
*DAY LOW-CARB DAY**

BREAKFAST:
- *1 Portion of Smoked Salmon Slices **OR**, Egg White Omelet (3-5 Egg Whites) with Cut Tomatoes*
- *1-2 Slices of Whole Wheat Toast, **(HALF* of Bread if still on Low-Carb)***
- *Small Fruit Bowl, **(NO EXOTIC Fruit*if still on Low-Carb)***
- *1-2 Glasses of Water*
- *Optional: Coffee or Tea*
- *1 Multivitamin Supplement*

MID-MORNING SNACK:
- *1 Low-Carb Protein Shake **OR**, 1 Fruit **(NON-EXOTIC if still on Low-Carb)***
- *1-2 Glasses of Water or Tea*

LUNCH:
- *1 Portion of Lean Stir-Fry with Chicken or Shrimp, lots of Veggies and **1 Portion of Brown Rice or Polenta (HALF PORTION* of Rice or Polenta if still on Low-Carb)***
- *2 Glasses of Water or Unsweetened Iced Tea*
- *OPTIONAL: Coffee*

MID AFTERNOON SNACK:

▶ *Low-Fat/Low-Sugar Bran Muffin* OR, 1 Orange, Peach or Banana* or other Fruit (switch to Normal-Carb)*

▶ *1-2 Glasses of Water*

▶ *Optional: Coffee or Tea*

DINNER:

▶ *Ground Turkey or Turkey Sausage Pasta: **FULL PORTION Pasta***, mixed with 1 portion of cooked lean Turkey Sausage OR ground Turkey, and a tomato sauce made of 100% natural cut tomatoes (caned or fresh), mixed with 1 tablespoon of Olive Oil and some natural spices, such as basil. OPTIONAL: add some non-fat Parmesan. It's a normal-carb Evening: **enjoy a piece of whole wheat bread* along** with some mixed fruits as a desert*

OR, LICENSE TO CHEAT:

▶ *Whatever you desire! But keep portions still as small as possible and choose ingredients as healthy as possible. Eat slowly, it will make you enjoy cheating food more and prevent overeating. Quality is still more important than Quantity, even when eating not 100% Healthy Meals. That said: ENJOY with no Regrets!*

Optional Night-Snack:

▶ ***Bowl of Melons or Pineapples* OR,** Hot Chocolate with Non-fat Milk or Soymilk*

SUNDAY EXAMPLE
= *NORMAL-CARB DAY / DAY OFF*

Sunday is fun day! I personally like to eat a "little less healthy as usual" breakfast on Sundays, which can even include some pancakes or a normal cereal for change. I also like to go to the Farmers Market and buy some fresh fruits. Since Sunday is a normal-carb day this includes lots of exotic fruit choices such as melons, oranges, and bananas. Further, almost every Sunday, I make sure to enjoy a non-fat Cafe Mocha together with 1-2 muffins or scones or a bagel. For lunch or dinner I might choose some delicious sushi and if I feel like I may even have some pizza, frozen yogurt, or another "empty calorie" food choice like ice cream. Sunday is a day-off your regular diet – especially if you made most of Saturday a low-carb day. If for whatever reason some days during your week turned into cheating, use Sunday to eat mostly healthy food, but make sure to eat more carbs no matter what since you do not want to start Monday with an empty or low-carb storage system but an all filled-up and replenished one. Only if it's full you can empty it again slowly. Also, as a reminder, if you are just starting Stage 1 of your Carb Cycle, start implementing healthier food choices into your diet during the first days and weeks in order to cleanse out your system of as much unhealthy food as possible. Then, when you switch to Stage 2, change to mostly healthy food choices. I promise you that you will feel the difference. Further, once your body is cleansed by eating new and healthier choices you make during weekdays, your metabolism can tolerate cheating on weekends much better. Whatever you decide to do in terms of the exact food choices on your cheating day, try to stop eating unhealthy food choices again towards the evening hours on Sunday. Sunday night is the time to still enjoy some healthy carbs like exotic Fruits, a nice Pasta Dinner, or any other healthy meal combination. But your next Carb Cycle is about to begin and it's time to go back to 100% as healthy as possible food choices.

CHAPTER 8

HOW TO EXERCISE WITH CARB CYCLE

Although my Carb Cycle Diet works without exercising, I strongly recommend you to combine it with Regular Physical Activity. Our bodies were made to be active and exercise. In fact, the human body thrives on activity. If we're not active, once we reach around 25 years of age, we gradually start losing muscle tissue, agility, and cardiovascular ability. As our muscle mass decreases, the risk of developing health problems such as osteoporosis, arthritis, and back pain increases. Further, muscles are the only tissue that burns both fat and carbohydrates, and plays a huge role in regulating your metabolism. Last but not least, the most important muscle in the human body – the heart – thrives on regular physical activity.

The benefits of exercising and being active in the 21st Century are endless, but unfortunately so are the options. There are countless exercise systems and programs available, from ones that promise you'll get into great shape without really doing much, and others that have you doing extreme, very high-intensity routines. The result is that most people are totally confused and overwhelmed as to what they should do when it comes to exercising. Personally, it makes me upset to see this all taking place since it either makes people afraid of exercising and/or wastes their time with unnecessary, potentially even dangerous techniques.

Now, while these very intense routines can work for some athletes and extreme sports enthusiasts, they typically don't work for the average person, especially in the long-term. The solution lies, as with dieting, in the past: Our Ancestors.

Thousands of years ago, we may have walked up to thirty miles per day. That's because we were living or working outside and were forced to be active. If we wanted to eat, we couldn't just head down to the nearest supermarket or the drive-thru. Instead we had to hunt and forage for our food. This often meant we ran after our prey, or ran from being somebody else's next meal. We simply didn't require extra activity because we were already getting enough. Well, not anymore!

These days, most of us have jobs and lifestyles that are sedentary. A walk to the coffee machine is about the only consistent exercise most people get on a daily basis. It's estimated that we engage in 90% less physical activity today than our great-grandparents did at the turn of the last century. In addition, our diets have deteriorated to where we eat far too much processed food that is full of sugar, fat, chemicals, additives, and other bad ingredients.

Obviously, our world has changed, and that's mostly a good thing. We don't need to walk thirty miles per day looking for our next meal, and not having enough food is rarely a problem. The real problem is that while our world has changed, our bodies haven't. They still behave upon the assumption that you're going to be moving around a lot and that you'll be eating healthy foods. However, as discussed, that's not really happening, at least not by itself anymore.

Now, more than ever, we need to make sure we give our body those daily physical activity impulses, as well as to start to eat food again the way nature intended. We need to do this if we are going to fight new age diseases such as obesity successfully, and live a long, healthy, and happy life.

THE BASIC THREE ELEMENTS OF EXERCISING

There are three Elements that make a balanced Exercise Routine:

1) TONING =
Sculpting & Strengthening

2) CARDIOVASCULAR =
Endurance & Fat Burning

3) STRETCHING =
Flexibility & Agility

GETTING STARTED

The biggest problem I see is when people jump from doing nothing at all in the way of exercise and physical activity, right into working out in an extreme manner. If you are not used to exercise you should really start step-by-step and ideally lose some body weight first before starting any high intensity workout program.

I know my view might appear too simple in a world full of fancy fitness routines, but until you are already at a healthy weight, I strongly advise you to begin working out slowly. Start by taking fitness walks every day and doing some simple toning exercises for at least one month. Build your stamina & strength slowly – step by step – using only your body weight and lighter weights on machines. Make sure to start doing some simple stretching exercises every day as well. I'm convinced that following this advice is the right way to start a physical exercise routine for probably 80% of the population.

If you are new to exercising or haven't done it in a while, I suggest you to do the following:

TONING:

2-4 times per week for 15 minutes for the first month, then gradually build up to 30-60 minutes

When it comes to toning and strengthening, the quality of the movements you do is more important than the quantity of time you spend working out. Correct, simple strengthening exercises and slow movements are the best way to go, especially for the first weeks of your exercise routine. A light total-body routine with simple equipment such as dumbbells or rubber bands or at the gym with basic machines works best for the first few weeks. After you build a foundation like this, you can step by step build it up to a more intense program which includes more machines and exercise equipment, along with more intense techniques and heavier weights.

CARDIO:

1-2 times daily for 15 minutes for the first month, then gradually build up to 1-2 times daily for 30-60 minutes

When it comes to Cardio, the longer and less intense the better. One of the reasons for this is that fat is burned most efficiently if the intensity is moderate but therefore can be done longer and more often. That is why a daily brisk walk, bike ride, or any other fun activity is an excellent cardio choice, especially for the first couple of weeks. After that it can be built up to more intense and advanced cardio options. Usually, after a few weeks of moderate exercising not only does the body get used to exercising, but also the first weight loss success makes any more intense cardio option much more doable. For example, I do not think anybody who is overweight or out of shape should go jogging right away. The stress is just too much for the body. After a couple of weeks of fitness walking and healthy nutrition which result in an already reduced body weight it's much easier and healthier to start more intense cardio options.

STRETCHING:

Every day for 5-15 minutes

Rule number one: Stretching means "relaxing" – not flexing or forcing any movements or positions! A good stretching routine can be done anytime and everywhere, at least once daily for 5-15 Minutes. Stretching is also ideally combined with exercising, either as a warm-up and/or cool-down.

Other great times to stretch include when you're at work, in front of the TV, whenever you get stiff, and before going to bed. I personally like to stretch a little before going to bed in order to release any stiffness in my body for a healthy, recuperating sleep.

SETTING UP YOUR INDIVIDUAL EXERCISE ROUTINE

Setting up your personal, individual activity routine depends on your individual lifestyle and schedule. The goal is to be flexible and make time whenever you can in order to work on all three elements of exercising as much as necessary.

There are many simple ways to combine your workouts. For example, you can work on your strength on Monday, Tuesday, Thursday, and Friday by performing toning exercises using your own bodyweight, or by lifting weights. Ideally every day you can work on cardio by taking walks, bike rides, and doing other aerobic activities. Even better, you can do a 15-30 minute cardio session every day along with some additional toning and stretching exercises.

Once you become more used to exercising, you can start splitting up your workouts into two or even three short ones per day. For example, you could work out 15 minutes in the morning, and then another 15 minutes in the afternoon or evening. You can even try squeezing in few minutes of exercise here and there throughout the day. The advantage of splitting up your exercising into several smaller sessions is that it helps boost your metabolism.

Additionally and maybe most important: move your body whenever possible in your normal daily activities! Take the stairs instead of the elevator. Park your car a little further away than you normally would when you drive somewhere. Get up to change the channel instead of using the remote. This additional activity will pay off by making your metabolism run faster and smoother all day long.

CROSS TRAINING

You can also combine all three fitness elements into one complete total body workout. For example do 5-15 minutes of weight training, followed by 10-20 minutes of cardio, finishing with 7-10 minutes of stretching. All in just 20-45 minutes! If you do this 2-4 times per week, you will see a big difference in your general health, fitness, and weight loss goals. The workout length and intensity depends on the Carb Cycle Stage and Exercise Level you are on. Again, always use common sense and build up your way slowly but steadily.

If you decide to combine your workouts, always do your toning workout first followed by your cardio workout. This way you will burn fat faster and more efficiently. That's because your body will already be warmed up. Your body has to "heat up" for 10-15 minutes in order to burn fat optimally, so always keep that in mind.

On my website, **WWW.CARBCYCLE.COM**, I'm soon going to provide more information & free downloads all around exercising. Also, as mentioned before, I will be offering 3 Stages from Starter to Advanced, leading you day-by-day through your Carb Cycle *and* Exercise Routine. However, make sure to start with these simple exercise rules and you are on your way to get and stay in great shape for life.

THE BEST TIME TO EXERCISE

People often ask me, "When is the best time to exercise?" The answer is that there is no wrong time to exercise. If you want to do it in the middle of the night, go ahead. Any time is a good time to exercise, as long as you do it. There is only one exception to this. Don't exercise right after you eat. Wait at least 30-60 minutes in order to give your body some time to digest your meal. However, if I had to choose the best time to workout, it would be first thing in the morning on an empty stomach, other than lots of water and perhaps some black coffee.

There are several reasons why the morning is the best time to work out. It will give your metabolism a boost that lasts throughout the day, it increases mental acuity, giving you more brainpower, and most important, because you haven't eaten yet, your body is naturally forced to burn fat faster. The only rule is to drink plenty of water before, during, and after being active, and to make sure you eat a healthy breakfast right after being active.

I find that the best activities for a morning workout are simply walking or biking outside in nature. I usually ride my bike for 5-10 minutes to a nearby park or garden where I walk around for 10—20 minutes. Then, I ride my bike back home. If I don't have my bike available, walking alone is great and certainly does the job.

Another option is to find some stairs and walk up and down a few times before resuming your normal walk. You can even do some toning movements between going up and down the stairs. Additionally, speed up your pace every 3-5 minutes for a few seconds or so in order to get an extra kick, then go back to your normal pace. Be flexible and creative when it comes to being active – there are many ways to exercise by using just a pair of sneakers, which by the way I always keep in my car.

If you want to visit the gym or do toning at home first thing in the morning, that's great too. Use the same rules for all kinds of exercising. Always start with a little bit of stretching, use common sense, and don't do anything your body can't handle. Remember, when it comes to being active, anything you do is better than nothing.

THE THREE DAILY ACTIVITY LEVELS:

Here are three daily activity levels you can choose from to create your own exercise program. They fit together with the 3 Carb Cycle Stages I talked about in Chapter 6. Keep in mind though that Carb Cycle Stage 3 and Exercise Level 3 are for people who really want to maximize their weight loss results over a certain period of time or for competitive athletes. For anybody new to a fit and healthy lifestyle, it's important to start with Level 1 for the first 30 days, and for anybody who wants to stay fit and healthy, feel and look great Level 2 is usually enough. My advice is that you focus on Level 1 and 2, and thereafter decide if Level 3 is appropriate for you and your fitness goals.

EXERCISE LEVEL 1

INTENSITY:
STARTER

DURATION:
15-30 MINUTES DAILY

▶ *EXERCISE 1 X DAILY FOR 15-30 MINUTES,* **OR**
▶ *2 X 15 MINUTES DAILY IN ORDER TO* **SUPPORT** *YOUR DIET RESULTS & GET USED TO EXERCISING SLOWLY*

<u>**Starter Example:**</u> Walk every day for 15-30 minutes and add a simple toning routine into that workout 2-3 times per week. Stretch whenever you can, preferably 2-4 times per week for 7-15 minutes. Another option is to workout 10 minutes in the morning, and 10 minutes in the evening.

EXERCISE LEVEL 2

INTENSITY:
INTERMEDIATE

DURATION:
30-60 MINUTES DAILY

- ► *EXERCISE 1 X DAILY FOR 30-60 MINUTES,* **OR**
- ► *2 X DAILY FOR 15-30 MINUTES TO* **OPTIMIZE** *YOUR DIET RESULTS*

Intermediate Example: Do some toning or combined toning and cardio for 15-30 minutes in the morning and another session in the evening. Or do a 30-60 minute workout once per day, whenever you can make that much time. Stretch out a little before, between, or after your workouts.

EXERCISE LEVEL 3

INTENSITY:
ADVANCED

DURATION:
MORE THAN 60 MINUTES DAILY

▶ *EXERCISE UP TO 3 X DAILY FOR 30-60 MINUTES THROUGH AM/MID-DAY/PM WORKOUTS IN ORDER TO **MAXIMIZE** YOUR DIET RESULTS FOR A CERTAIN PERIOD OF TIME*

Advanced Example: Perform up to three workouts per day, one in the morning, the next at midday, and the last in the evening. For example, take a fast walk for 20-30 minutes first thing in the morning on an empty stomach, then, at midday, do some toning for 15-45 minutes, then, in the evening do some more cardio for 30-60 minutes. This is really going to maximize your fat burning, and will help you shape up as fast as possible, especially if you do it in combination with Carb Cycle. However, it's not necessary unless you really want to push the limits and it's **NOT** for starters. It's for advanced fitness enthusiasts only. **I will talk more about this and some "Advanced Carb Cycle" Techniques in Chapter 9.**

In order to prevent your metabolism from slowing down, make sure to always drink plenty of water before, during, and after any exercise. Also, never workout for more than 60 Minutes at a time, unless you're doing a very low intensity hike, bike ride, or walk.

In closing this chapter, keep in mind that whatever exercise routine you choose, the goal is that you get in shape and stay that way for life. Just like your diet, this is not a sprint, but a journey. Do your minimal daily activity and choose it wisely. Whether it is sports, exercise DVD's, fun activities, boot camps, pilates, or anything else, there are hundreds of ways to combine activities in order to fully utilize the three basic components of exercising. The key is to find and commit to a program that you can follow. Make it a daily habit to schedule time to be active into your calendar, just like a business meeting. Personally, I believe that nothing beats a daily brisk fitness walk, along with some basic toning and stretching exercises to get and stay in shape for life!

Remember, solutions, not excuses are key. Never forget that exercising doesn't take time, but *GIVES* you time, because you are going to live longer and are less likely to become ill if you do it regularly.

NOTE: This is mainly a diet book, and the focus is on the Carb Cycle Nutrition System. For more exercise information log on to **WWW.CARBCYCLE.COM** where I will soon talk more about exercising and explain more details including videos and pictures of all the most effective exercises, techniques, and tricks all around working out.

CHAPTER 9

ADVANCED
CARB CYCLE

TEMPORARILY MAXIMIZING THE INTENSITY OF YOUR CARB CYCLE

Before I start this section please let me give you a <u>*WARNING:*</u> **Do not go on any Extreme or Advanced Carb Cycle without already being used to the Normal Carb Cycle for at least 2 months, as well as having been exercising for at least 2 months by getting gradually used to a fair amount of daily physical activity.**

Any beginners should first go through Stage 1 and Stage 2 of the Basic Carb Cycle I wrote about in earlier chapters. In case you are an athlete or want to take the Carb Cycle concept to the maximum, make sure to use common sense, and if necessary consult with your doctor. For anybody who is not already pretty lean and fit and already has a body fat percentage of 15% or less, it doesn't really make sense to go beyond the first two stages of the basic 50% Carb Cycle. Advanced Carb Cycle can help you break a barrier from lean to extra lean, but is not necessary to achieve a lean and healthy body. Until you have that, stick to Stage 1 and Stage 2, although of course you can keep reading this chapter in order to be ready in a few weeks or months and understand the Carb Cycle System even better. You can absolutely skip Stage 3 and stick to Stage 1 and 2 which are all you need to get a lean and healthy body. That said, Advanced Carb Cycle can be a lot of fun since it is the first EVER outline of how to really achieve that extra lean "Fitness Model" look in the most simple, yet effective way possible.

As you first come to learn about my Carb Cycle System, you might ask how much more you could eliminate your "Basic Carbs" on your depleting days than the recommended 50%. Well, that all depends on how active you are and what your goals are. Although I've mapped out a fairly specific schedule for the Normal Carb Cycle Program, you can further fine-tune this to accommodate your individual lifestyle, weight goals, and activity levels. That is once you are ready and want to achieve peak conditioning.

As you know by now, the Main Carb Cycle Schedule has you reducing all Basic Carbs = Grains and Starches by 50% along with limiting Exotic Fruits on low-carb days. However, once you follow the Carb Cycle for a couple of months and complete Stages 1 and 2, there are further adjustments possible based on how active you want to be, and what goals beyond being healthy and looking fit you might like to achieve. Once you become more familiar with the Carb Cycle, it's fairly simple to fine-tune the amount of carbs you're reducing on your low-carb days based on how much you might want to additionally chisel and trim down. Here are the two main ways to do this:

First, you can balance your Carb Cycle results by changing the amount of exercise you do. If you're planning on exercising every day or are extraordinarily active, you can eat some more carbs on your low-carb days. The 50% rule is always the baseline and the best way to start for the first 30-60 days. However, if you are an "Advanced Carb Cycler" so to say you can always adjust this level up or down depending on your circumstances. On the other hand, if you are not exercising at all (which I do not recommend!) you can temporarily try cutting your carbs by 75% on those days of zero or limited physical activity. Once you get used to cycling your carbs, you will see that all this minor but highly effective adjustments are really simple to do. Keep in mind that the cycle itself is the most important thing, not the exact percentage of carbs you cut. Our ancestors surely didn't count carb percentages and were still able to use their carb storage areas most effectively by always being in the "Carb Cycle Zone."

Second, you can change the intensity of your Carb Cycle based on your trim down goals. In fact, your ultimate fitness goals are a great way to determine how much to cut your carbs on low-carb days. As a rule of thumb, if your goal is to lose those last stubborn few pounds of fat around your waist or love handles, then cut your carbs by 50% - 75% on your carb-restricted days PLUS exercise as much as you can. If you're losing weight too fast, just increase the amount of carbs you eat on your low-carb days slightly, and if you're not losing weight fast enough, decrease them slightly.

Whatever intensity level you choose, *NEVER* cut your carbs for more than 75% on your low-carb days, and always re-load them normally every 3rd or 4th day for at least one day.

Again, for a normal, basic Carb Cycle which always should make the majority of your Cycles, the best number to cut your carbs is by 50%, as there's no way you can go wrong by sticking to this.

ADVANCED CARB CYCLE TECHNIQUES FOR ULTIMATE RESULTS

The information I am about to share with you is basically the way I used my Carb Cycle to achieve peak conditioning and win all my Mr. World Fitness Titles in the late 1990's and early 2000. There is no need to switch to these high intensity levels unless you are already pretty lean and in great overall fitness shape. Once you are, the following information will give you another optional kick, and will get you into the best shape of your life in terms of being really lean and ripped. Not just fit and healthy shape – but even athletic, six-pack – or eight-pack - World Fitness shape.

In order to really lose weight fast (something I *DO NOT* recommend), get rid of those stubborn last few pounds, or to temporarily lower your body fat percentage below 12 %, you can exercise more and/or cut your carbs for up to 75% daily on low-carb days. However, as mentioned, always use common sense. Whenever you either feel too weak, or reach a totally empty storage level too quickly, then eat some more carbs and reduce the amount of exercise you're doing or the amount of carbs you are depleting. Also, never skip the carb re-loading phase, and eat higher amounts of carbs on your normal-carb days, which are probably Wednesdays and Sundays.

Now, whenever you want to push your results a little, you can make whole Saturday an optional low-carb day as well. I always recommend clients who want to maximize their results to do this. However, having said this, remember, you need carbs in order to exercise and for your metabolism to function properly, and once your storage is empty it's really imperative you reload them again very soon.

By the way, if you don't have a feeling for when your carbs are empty yet, or you want to be absolutely sure, you can buy ketosis sticks. I never used them much and prefer to go by the way I feel. As long as you empty your carb storage slowly and steadily over a 2-3 days period, you'll be fine. Also, once you reached your weight goal and just want to maintain your weight, it's enough to cut your carbs by only 50% or even less again on low-carb days. Always keep in mind that optimum results don't occur when you're burned out or rushing beyond reason. There is a difference between working hard, and working too hard. Work hard but also rest hard. That's definitely a motto that applies to Advanced Carb Cycle.

Another way to speed up results is to skip your cheating meals completely for a few weeks and just eat healthy, natural foods and carbs on Sundays, just like you would on Wednesday. The most important reminder is to respect the main Carb Cycle rules, be flexible and rational, and use common sense. Doing this will ensure your success with my Carb Cycle Diet, no matter what intensity level you are going to follow.

On another note, if you lose weight in stages, don't worry. I actually like to hear this. Losing 2-3 pounds, staying there a few days, then maybe even sometimes gain a pound back, and then again losing more pounds is a much healthier way for the body to adjust and lose weight. Also, sometimes you might lose 3 pounds of fat and gain 3 pounds of muscle which results in no weight change or even weight gain. This is normal and okay. In order not to drive yourself crazy, try not to weigh yourself too often, perhaps 1-2 times per week, and do it at the same time of the day. The sizes of your clothes and the mirror are sometimes a much better way to determine your ongoing success instead of weighing yourself constantly.

COMBINING ACTIVITY WITH ADVANCED CARB CYCLE FOR MAXIMUM RESULTS

The amount of carbs that you eliminate on your Advanced Carb Cycle depleting days should be in balance with your activity and exercise level and goals. This all depends on how much you want to invest beyond the normal recommended daily activity level, and the normal 50% reduction on low-carb days. Please note that I use the word invest, as this extra effort and time is an investment and great effort, but one that WILL pay off and optimize your results. Whenever you want to maximize your results, I suggest you do a minimum of 30-60 minutes of daily exercise. Again, if you are fairly new to daily exercising, a simple 15-30 minute daily walk can be enough for the first weeks. Always start slowly and give your body time to adapt. From there you can slowly add time and intensity as appropriate. However, the higher your fitness and weight-loss goals are, the more you might want to work out, up to 1-2 hours per day, ideally split into shorter, but more frequent work outs. I suggest you increase your exercise amount and intensity week by week by no more than 10-20 minutes at a time. Be patient, but persistent and give your body time to adapt. You want to get it in shape, not break it.

The easiest way to combine and adjust your Advanced Carb Cycle with exercise is to use the 3 basic exercise intensity levels I talked about in the activity chapter. You can easily choose and switch between them anytime. The only thing that changes when you are on an Advanced Carb Cycle is that you might work out more but still cut your Carbs more as well. Or - especially in case you sometimes do not work out at all – reduce them temporarily for a little bit more on such no activity days. Let me explain further:

Exercise Level 1 "Starter" is perfect for beginners, as well as for maintaining any achieved success. It should be the minimum amount of activity you do. Exercise Level 2 "Intermediate," is a healthy medium, and Exercise Level 3 "Advanced," is for more enthusiastic people or even athletes who desire to lose weight faster or achieve higher goals then just being fit and healthy.

These 3 Daily Activity Levels from chapter eight do not only determine how much you should be active every day when starting your Carb Cycle. Further, they also help you decide how much you can raise or lower your carbs once you are on an Advanced Carb Cycle Routine.

ADVANCED CARB CYCLE ACTIVITY ADJUSTMENTS:

ACTIVITY LEVEL 1:
LOW

- Being Active and working out the minimum of 15-30 minutes per day or less
- **Advanced Carb Cycle Adjustment:** Reduce your basic carb intake by up to 75% on low-carb days

ACTIVITY LEVEL 2:
MEDIUM

- Being active and working out up to 60 minutes per day, split into 1-2 workouts
- **Advanced Carb Cycle Adjustment:** Reduce your basic carb intake by 50-75% on your low-carb days

ACTIVITY LEVEL 3:
HIGH

- Being active and working out more than 60 minutes per day, split into 2 or more workouts
- **Advanced Carb Cycle Adjustment:** Reduce your basic carb intake by 25-50 % on low-carb days

Don't forget that ultimately it all depends on whether you want to lose or maintain weight. If you want to chisel down and lean out to the max, you can exercise more than 60 minutes and still cut your "Basic Carbs" by even 75% on your low-carb days. However, always reload them every 3 days and eat enough to still have adequate energy. As a reminder, and I know I said this a thousand times already: *NEVER EVER* **cut out carbs completely, not even on your lowest carb days on an Advanced Carb Cycle Program.** On the other hand, once you have achieved your ideal weight, exercising will allow you to eat some extra carbs without gaining weight. It's the old rule of nature we discussed before; eat what you burn and burn what you eat!

You can also switch between the three basic intensity levels from week-to-week, or even day-to-day. For example, if you want to workout more often during certain days of your week, let's say on Saturday and Sunday, just adjust your diet and exercise routine from level 1 or 2 to level 3 for the weekend. You can do the same if you don't exercise for 1-2 days, just switch from level 3 to level 2 or 1. There are no limitations and this is the great thing about my system. Once you understand it, it is very simple and easy to adjust, all while being highly accurate and effective regarding how your body will react to what you eat and how much you exercise.

I know I said this before, but want to emphasize again that **these techniques are for Advanced Carb Cycle Users only.** No beginner should worry about this and try to adjust the Carb Cycle beyond the Basic 2 Stages and the normal 50% rule. Still, if you are reading this, it's great to know that you have further options to play with once you are on the Carb Cycle for a couple of months. On another note, this just reminds me of a favorite quote of mine I'm using for years: **Play with your Carbs instead of letting them play with you!** That quote fits perfectly to the normal Carb Cycle and definitely continues with Advanced Carb Cycle!

SOME HIGH-INTENSITY CARB CYCLE TRICKS FOR ATHLETES AND/OR MAXIMUM RESULTS

Once you are down to a certain body fat percentage and temporarily want to push your limits with the more Advanced Carb Cycle Levels I wrote about in this chapter, here are some additional high-intensity Tricks, Tips, and Reminders:

▶ **Intensity Level:** As explained above, the more you exercise and the more you cut your carbs on low-carb days, the leaner you will get. However, there is *NO* need to do this unless you are already in great shape which means a body fat percentage of below 12-15%. If you are there and want to get in even better shape, exercising up to 2-3 times per day (but never for more than 60 Minutes at a time), and cutting your carbs for up to 75 Percent on your low-carb days is an option. Whenever you are on an Advanced Carb Cycle, make sure to eat some extra healthy fat on your low-carb days and to reload your carb storage accordingly every 3rd or at least 4th day no matter what. Further, even on the highest intensity Advanced Carb Cycle: *NEVER EVER* cut out carbs completely from your meals!

▶ **Cut out Dairy (any milk products) for a few weeks:** If you are already lean that will make you look even leaner. I usually stopped eating dairy products for 3-6 weeks before I competed or had a photo shoot, since any milk product – even nonfat – contains lactose and can potentially smooth out that ultra-thin skin "look" you might desire. The same rule applies for any manufactured protein products such as whey protein powders or protein shakes, although I would suggest you only cut these for the last 1-2 weeks before your competition or special day you want to look the most chiseled and toned. Cutting milk products only makes sense temporarily, as I just described, or if you are lactose intolerant. I personally love milk too much and there's no reason to cut milk out, but rather enjoy it in moderation and its fat-free versions. Also, unless your body fat percentage is very low you won't see a difference, so wait till you are rather lean before considering temporarily sacrificing any milk products.

▶ **Counting Grams:** There is no need to count the grams of carbs you are eating on a normal Carb Cycle program. However, if you switch to a high-intensity Advanced Carb Cycle Level, a good rule of thumb is to eat anywhere between 50-150 grams of carbs on your low-carb days, and anywhere between 200-400 grams on your normal-carb days. I personally always ate more than 75 Grams even on my lowest-carb days – especially since I was always physically active. I suggest not to go lower than 75 grams if you are male, and no lower than 50 grams if you are female. These are the maximal low-carb day numbers even when following an Advanced Carb Cycle Diet. Another rule of thumb is to go by your bodyweight: on low-carb days eat as low as 0.5 grams per pound, on normal-carb days as much as 1.5 to 2 grams per pound. This means a person weighing 200 lbs. can go to as low as 100 grams of carbs on a low-carb day. Again, I usually **DO NOT** go by these numbers but by how I feel, how active I am, and how fast I want to either lose or maintain weight and fat. Common sense is the most important rule, but since this chapter is for Advanced Carb Cycling, I wanted to make sure to share these numbers with you.

▶ **Work hard on your weights:** This is the time to do short but high-intensity workouts when it comes to toning & strength. This will further deplete your carbs on your low-carb days and put your muscles into a mode where they can't wait to load carbs again. However, when it comes to cardio – mostly work on a medium to low-intensity level and for longer times. The lower your body fat percentage gets, the more your body is holding on to your fat reserves. Fat burning requires heat, oxygen, and water – the best way to provide this is to do cardio for longer periods of time with less intensity and lots of water.

▶ **Ketosis:** Although you never want to stay there too long, taking your Carb Cycle to the highest level might include that you get close to or even reach Ketosis - the state of a completely emptied carb storage - and stay there for a little while, but never too long. Using Ketosis Sticks – available in every pharmacy or even on Amazon.com - to measure this makes sure you never stay there too long. I would not recommend staying there for more than a few hours. If you ever reach Ketosis too early before you start re-loading your carbs again – reduce your workout intensity a little or eat slightly more carbs on your low-carb days. Remember, optimum fat burning, along with a high metabolic rate occurs "while" you are slowly and steadily depleting and re-loading your carb storage, but never staying neither depleted or full for too long.

▶ **Best Food Choices to Maximize Your Results:** This is the time to focus on simple, "one-ingredient" Food Choices. For Carbs, I would stick to Oatmeal, Brown Rice, Potatoes, and Sweet Potatoes. For Protein, Lean Poultry, and Fish along with Egg Whites. For Fat, use Olive Oil and Nuts. Vegetables and Salad are always good but skip any high fructose/exotic fruits. Stay with apples and pears. This is not something I suggest to keep for a long period of time, but if you want to chisel down and temporary get in extra lean shape it's what has worked for me. However, this way of eating requires the most discipline and motivation, just be aware of this before you think about starting it.

▶ **Lots of Water:** Drink up to 2 Gallons per day if you work out a lot. Also, 1-3 black coffees and/or Green Teas are great to drink and will help keep your metabolism running high, especially right before your physical activity segments.

▶ **Multivitamin:** At any given point NEVER skip a decent Multivitamin Supplement when following an Advanced Carb Cycle Routine. For any intense fitness routine, I would further suggest taking the following supplements: 1 Vitamin E Supplement, 1 Calcium-Magnesium Supplement, and 1 Vitamin C Supplement.

▶ **Empty Stomach AM Workouts:** Whenever you can, especially on your low-carb days, implement some "first thing in the morning" physical activity on an empty stomach. Being active that way, the body can access and burn fat much more efficiently and quickly. Besides, it's the perfect way to kick-start your metabolism for the day. Even a simple 15 minute walk can do wonders and if done 4-5 times per week will make a huge difference in your fat burning results along with the Carb Cycle. I personally do some empty stomach physical activity almost every morning. Here's three simple rules to keep in mind whenever you can implement empty stomach workouts: 1) Drink plenty of water right after waking up, 2) Take a fast walk for 15-30 minutes, and 3) Eat a healthy breakfast right after.

▶ **A Note for Competitive Athletes in any Sport:** If you are a competitive athlete, make sure to load your carbs 1-2 days "before" your competition date. For example, if your competition is on Saturday, I would suggest you to lower your carbs on Mon, Tues, and Wed – then load them on Thur and Fri. This way has two major benefits: 1) You are sure you go "into" your competition with an "all-filled" carb storage system, ready & full the night before the competition. 2) Your body will temporarily most likely hold even more carbs this way, because whenever you first deplete your carbs and then load them, your storage can temporarily store more carbs right after. This is how I originally discovered the Carb Storage in the late 80's and then fine-tuned the Carb Cycle over years and years of trials and effort. However, everybody can just deplete carbs by avoiding them and load them by eating lots of them, but unless you accordingly and slowly lower your storage before for the exact amount of time I taught you in this book, you'll never get the most out of your carb storage potential. Coming from weeks and months of doing a normal Carb Cycle though – all you have to do is adjust it slightly as I just described before your "big" competition day.

This concludes the information around "Advanced Carb Cycle" for the moment. I will definitely talk about this in more detail in the future – especially since more and more "Carb Cycle Enthusiasts" might soon want to get those chiseled, six-pack bodies.

Look for more information on WWW.CARBCYCLE.COM soon!

CHAPTER 10

CARB CYCLE
FOR LIFE

MAINTAINING YOUR LEAN AND HEALTHY BODY

By now you've learned why diets work and why they don't. You've also learned how to eat carbs without storing them as fat, and that my Carb Cycle Diet is the most powerful and most rational way to lose and control weight. It combines all of the advantages of a low-carb diet, but doesn't have any of the disadvantages, like dramatically slowing down your metabolism. My Carb Cycle Diet only requires you to go low-carb with certain carbs for a few days. You get to eat carbs at all times. This makes my diet so much more effective and doable.

CARB CYCLE STAGE 4:

Once you went through Carb Cycle Stage 1 and 2 and optionally Stage 3 and attained your desired weight and all in shape dream body, Carb Cycle doesn't end there. I'll now show you how to **MAINTAIN** your perfect body once you have it. That is - so to say - actually Carb Cycle Stage 4! As I mentioned in the first chapters, any diet or fitness program should allow you to first achieve a lean and healthy body, as well as thereafter give you a method to **MAINTAIN IT FOR GOOD.**

In order to control and maintain your weight successfully FOR LIFE, you need to be aware that your body's metabolism is always in one of three zones: 1) *GAINING WEIGHT,* 2) *MAINTAINING WEIGHT,* or 3) *LOSING WEIGHT.*

LOSING WEIGHT:

In order to lose weight and burn fat, the Carb Cycle is the best option. As you know by now, carbs are the only food category you can and should adjust or re-arrange drastically to reach your weight-loss goals. That means you follow the plan that nature intended: using your storage of carbs constantly by loading and depleting it, eating the right carbs on the right cycle in order to simultaneously burn off any excess fat reserves.

As I explained in Chapter 9, once you are used to the normal Carb Cycle, you can temporarily adopt an "Advanced Carb Cycle" in order to even lose some more weight quickly and get in absolute peak condition.

However, once you've reached your desired weight, it's not necessary to continue with such intense carb cycles anymore. At this point you could change back to a less-intense carb cycle, or even a normal "moderation" diet in order to maintain your success. This would mean just eating good-carbs like you would on your normal-carb days. You can follow the common sense rule of "eat as much as you burn."

Nevertheless, there are two dangers whenever you switch to a moderation diet: 1) It is much more difficult to control and avoid being either too empty or full, and 2) your carb storage once again is "not" used or cycled to its full capacity!

Therefore, even though a moderation diet is acceptable when maintaining your weight, I personally prefer the Carb Cycle to maintain my weight. I do this by reducing my carbs by a moderate 25-50% on my low-carb days. I prefer this because my Carb Cycle Diet, even in a light cycle, has many advantages. To further clarify, here are the two options you can follow for a Carb Cycle for Life.

MAINTAINING WEIGHT – TWO OPTIONS:

In order to maintain any achieved ideal weight, keep cycling your carbs slightly OR switch back to eating them normally in moderation.

OPTION ONE:

To maintain your weight, either cycle your carbs in a very light way, or eat them in moderation at all times. Personally, I like to "slightly" cycle my carbs at all times. This allows me to constantly use my carb storage system in order to eat some extra carbs, and food, on my normal-carb days, without risking any weight gain. Remember, you should never eat carbs in high amounts, or bad carbs, on your carb-normal days unless you went low-carb the previous days. You ideally want to eat more carbs when your storage is empty, keeping carbs away from your fat cells.

This is why even when I want to maintain weight I still try to go into my weekends with at least a slightly depleted carb storage. I do this in order not to convert any excess carbs I might eat into fat, but instead store them in my liver and muscles. Then, starting on Monday, I will empty those "extra" stored carbs again. Usually cutting carbs by about 25-50% does this just perfectly while maintaining my weight.

OPTION TWO:

The other option to maintaining weight is to just eat carbs normally, but to do it in moderation. This is more like a normal moderation diet, which can potentially help you maintain your weight. However, this option can be very tricky. It is rather difficult to accurately monitor everything you eat and know if it's in harmony with what you're burning. It's more of a balancing act and requires more work than simply staying on the Carb Cycle.

Remember, any excess calories you potentially eat will be stored as fat, especially whenever if your carb storage areas aren't empty but already full. Therefore, be more careful if you want to maintain weight on a normal moderation diet.

However, the good thing is that whenever you might gain a little weight, just immediately switch back to my Carb Cycle Diet for a while. In any event, the Carb Cycle allows you to be in control of your weight at any given time.

CLOSING THOUGHTS

STAY FIT, STRONG, AND HEALTHY FOR LIFE

Life is a gift. Don't waste it. Make the right daily choices to be the best you can be in order to feel great, be happy, and live longer. Lead by example for your children, parents, brothers, sisters, friends, and even strangers. You have the power to change. Once you've made the decision in your heart, it is going to be easy. Enjoy life with optimum health and energy to its fullest potential. Take action now, for yourself and the ones you love!

It takes two things to get and stay in shape and be healthy. **First, you need to know how, and second, you need to do it**. Well, this book has definitely taught you how, so now it's time for you to take action. **Become the master of your health, well-being, and happiness – *THE MASTER OF YOUR LIFE*.**

I like to finish this book with one of my favorite quotes: "**A Person that is fit and healthy has a million wishes – a Person that is unfit and sick has but one!**" Choose to be fit and healthy now and for the rest of your life, and may all your other wishes and dreams become a reality too!

Eat on the right cycle, be active, and live with respect and integrity towards yourself and other people. This is what life is all about!

Yours in Optimum Fitness,

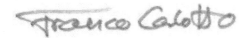

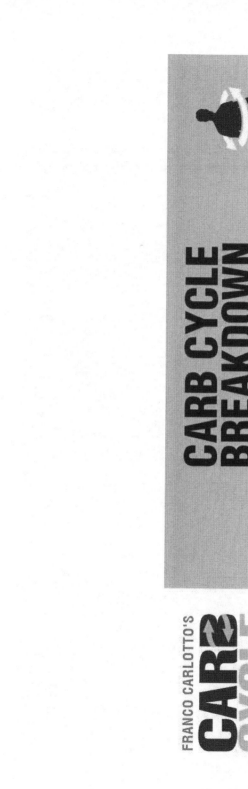

CARB CYCLE BREAKDOWN

FRANCO CARLOTTO'S
CARB CYCLE

THE BODY'S NATURAL CARB STORAGE SYSTEM

Your body can actually store carbs in your muscles and liver. The goal is to never have that storage constantly full or empty, but instead cycle it. By first depleting it, *(what takes about 2-3 days)* and then loading it again *(what takes about 1-2 days)*, you make sure that your carb storage never overflows (what turns carbs into fat) and that your metabolism never slows down (that's what happens when you stay on a constant low-carb diet). With the Carb Cycle, you are constantly burning fat while keeping your energy levels high. All while feeling great and losing weight.

Your body can actually store carbs

RULE:
Depleting your Storage takes 2-3 days, loading it takes 1-2 days

Too many or too little carbs make you fat:

If you are eating too many carbs & overfill your storage: Carbs turn into fat.

If you are constantly too low on carbs: Your body's metabolism slows down & protects it's fat depot.

The Solution

Start Using Your Carb Storage and *Cycle Your Carbs twice weekly* to burn off Fat

THE SOLUTION: CYCLE YOUR CARBS CONSTANTLY

Monday, Tuesday, Thursday, Friday, and daytime of Saturday you are eating low-carb and draining your carb storage like a cell-phone battery or kitchen sink by eating half of your normal Basic Carbs (Grains and Starches) and minimize Exotic Fruits. Wednesday, Saturday evening, and Sunday you are reloading your carbs by eating and enjoying all carbs normally. This is the most-effective weekly Carb Cycle which you can repeat again and again, and therefore finally control your weight for life.

CARB CYCLE FOOD RULES

The Food Rules for Carb Cycle are as simple as this:

CATEGORY	NORMAL-CARB DAY	LOW-CARB DAY
Protein	3-5 Servings Per Day	3-5 Servings Per Day
Carbohydrates: Basic (Grains & Starches)	Eat Normally	Cut by 50%
Carbohydrates: Vegetables & Legumes	2-4 Servings Per Day	2-4 Servings Per Day
Carbohydrates: Northern Fruits	2-4 Servings Per Day	2-4 Servings Per Day
Carbohydrates: Exotic Fruits	Eat Normal	Avoid or eat sparingly
Fat	In Moderation	In Moderation

WWW.CARBCYCLE.COM

FRANCO CARLOTTO'S

CARB CYCLE

PORTION SIZES & GOOD FOOD CHOICES

PORTION SIZES:

PROTEIN

One portion is about the size of your palm (without the fingers), except of protein powder, which is denser (usually 1 scoop is enough). If you eat fish, a portion size can be a little bigger = 1-2 times your palm.

CARBOHYDRATES

1. BASIC CARBS (Grains & Starches): One portion is about 1 times your palm size (without fingers)
2. VEGETABLES & LEGUMES: One portion is about 1-2 handfuls
3. FRUITS: One portion is about ½ to 1 of your palm size

FAT

One Portion of Nuts and Seeds: A Small Handful
One Portion of Oils: 1-2 Tablespoons
One Portion of Almond or Peanut Butter: 1-2 Teaspoons

GOOD FOOD CHOICES ARE:

PROTEIN

- Fish (Salmon, Haddock, Halibut, Tuna, etc.)
- Egg Whites (or substitutes)
- Lean Poultry (Chicken, Turkey, Ostrich)
- Lean Red Meat
- Shrimp, Lobster, Crab
- Tofu (& other Lean Soy Products)
- Nonfat or Lowfat Dairy Products (Cottage Cheese, Yogurt, Milk, etc.)
- Protein Shakes & Bars (low-carb = less than 200 Calories)
- Nuts (such as Almonds and Peanuts also contain Protein)

BASIC CARBS

- Oatmeal, Barley, Quinoa, etc.
- Brown Rice, Wild Rice,
- Rice Cakes, etc.
- Potatoes, Sweet Potatoes, etc.
- Whole Wheat Bread and
- Crackers
- Pasta
- Beans
- Corn
- Cereal (sugar-free!)
- Any Grain & Wheat Products

VEGETABLES/LEGUMES

- Broccoli
- Asparagus
- Squash & Pumpkin Varieties
- Zucchini
- Tomatoes
- Spinach
- Mushrooms
- Red, Yellow, Green Peppers
- Cauliflower
- Green Beans & Peas
- Salads, Celery, Cabbage, etc.

NORTHERN FRUITS

- Apples
- Pears
- Strawberries
- Blueberries
- Blackberries
- Grapes
- Raspberries
- Plums
- Cherries
- Etc.

EXOTIC FRUITS

- Bananas
- Grapefruits
- Oranges
- Pineapples
- Melons
- Papayas
- Mangos
- Nectarines
- Etc.

FAT

- Olive Oil
- Canola Oil
- Flax Seed Oil
- Avocado
- Olives
- Almonds & Peanuts
- Almond or Peanut Butter
- Sunflower Seeds
- Omega-3 Fats (Fish or Vegetable Oils)
- Other natural Nuts & Seeds

CARB
CYCLE

WEEKLY PLAN

		MONDAY & TUESDAY LOW-CARB DAYS	WEDNESDAY NORMAL-CARB DAY

BREAKFAST		• Portion Protein
		• HALF Portion Basic Carbs
		• Portion NORTHERN Fruits
		  or Vegetables
		• Portion Healthy Fat
		• 1-2 Glasses Water
		• Optional: Coffee or Tea
		• Suggested: Multivitamin
			• Portion Protein
			• FULL Portion Basic Carbs
			• Portion ANY Fruits
			  or Vegetables
			• Portion Healthy Fat
			• 1-2 Glasses Water
			• Optional: Coffee or Tea
			• Suggested: Multivitamin

**MID-
MORNING
SNACK**
		• Protein/Healthy Fat/NORTHERN
		  Fruit Mix Snack
		• 1-2 Glasses of Water or Tea
			• Protein/ANY Fruit Mix
			  OR Healthy Carb Snack
			• 1-2 Glasses of Water or Tea

LUNCH		• Portion Protein • HALF Portion Basic Carbs • Portion Vegetables • Portion Healthy Fat • 1-2 Glasses of Water or Tea	• Portion Protein • FULL Portion Basic Carbs • Portion Vegetables • Portion Healthy Fat • 1-2 Glasses of Water or Tea

**MID-
AFTERNOON
SNACK**
		• Protein/Healthy Fat/NORTHERN
		  Fruit Mix
		• 1-2 Glasses of Water
		• Optional: Coffee or Tea
			• Protein/ANY Fruit Mix
			  OR Healthy Carb Snack
			• 1-2 Glasses of Water
			• Optional: Coffee or Tea

DINNER		• Portion Protein • HALF OR LESS Portion Basic Carbs • 1-2 Portions Vegetables & Salad • Portion Healthy Fat • Water or Tea	• Portion Protein • FULL Portion Basic Carbs • Portion Vegetables & Salad • Portion Healthy Fat • Water/Tea

**OPTIONAL
NIGHT
SNACK**
		• Light Protein Snack with
		  some Northern Fruit
		  OR healthy Fat
		• Good Night Tea
			• Light Protein Snack with
			  ANY FRUIT
			• Good Night Tea

WWW.CARBCYCLE.COM

THURSDAY & FRIDAY
LOW-CARB DAYS

- Portion Protein
- HALF Portion Basic Carbs
- Portion NORTHERN Fruits or Vegetables
- Portion Healthy Fat
- 1-2 Glasses Water
- Optional: Coffee or Tea
- Suggested: Multivitamin

- Protein/Healthy Fat/NORTHERN Fruit Mix Snack
- 1-2 Glasses of Water or Tea

- Portion Protein
- HALF Portion Basic Carbs
- Portion Vegetables
- Portion Healthy Fat
- 1-2 Glasses of Water or Tea

- Protein/Healthy Fat/NORTHERN Fruit Mix
- 1-2 Glasses of Water
- Optional: Coffee or Tea

- Portion Protein
- HALF OR LESS Portion Basic Carbs
- 1-2 Portions Vegetables & Salad
- Portion Healthy Fat
- Water or Tea

- Light Protein Snack with some Northern Fruit OR healthy Fat
- Good Night Tea

SATURDAY
HALF LOW/NORMAL-CARB DAY

- Portion Protein
- HALF Portion Basic Carbs
- Portion NORTHERN Fruits or Vegetables
- Portion Healthy Fat
- 1-2 Glasses Water
- Optional: Coffee or Tea
- Suggested: Multivitamin

- Protein/Fat/NORTHERN Fruit Mix Snack
- 1-2 Glasses of Water or Tea

- Portion Protein
- HALF (OR FULL) Portion Basic Carbs
- Portion Vegetables
- Portion Healthy Fat
- 1-2 Glasses of Water or Tea

- Protein/ANY Fruit Mix OR Healthy Carb Snack
- 1-2 Glasses of Water
- Optional: Coffee or Tea

- Portion Protein
- FULL Portion Basic Carbs
- Portion Vegetables & Salad
- Portion Healthy Fat
- Water/Tea

- Light Protein Snack with ANY FRUIT OR Healthy Carb Snack
- Good Night Tea

SUNDAY
NORMAL-CARB DAY

LICENSE TO CHEAT

Sunday is a Normal-Carb day and an optional day of diet and exercise rest. Eat anything you like, within reason.

Sunday is Fun Day where you can enjoy some of the "bad" carbs or food choices you stayed away from during the week. Of course if you don't feel like eating any bad food choices, then don't - that's even better!

Whatever you do make sure to load your carbs on Sundays, especially during the morning hours and daytime in order to start your next Carb Cycle on Monday with a filled-up Carb Storage.

Remember, the key to successfully implementing The Carb Cycle Method is to never stay low- or high-carb for too long, but exactly using your body's storage system in the right way:

1) Depleting carbs for no more or less than 2-3 days, then

2) Loading carbs for no more or less than 1-2 days!

NOTE: For more details including exact Food Choices, Portion Sizes, and Meal Combinations refer to the main Carb Cycle Book and Charts!

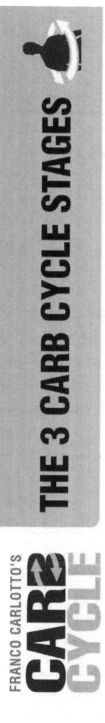

FRANCO CARLOTTO'S
CARB CYCLE

THE 3 CARB CYCLE STAGES

THERE ARE 3 CARB CYCLE STAGES FOR EVERYBODY

Each Stage is 30 days long:

Stage 1 is for Starters. Stage 2 is for Intermediate fitness levels. Stage 3 is for Advanced athletes and very seasoned fitness enthusiasts. For anybody new to a fit and healthy lifestyle, it's important and most efficient to start with Stage 1 then 2 for the first two months.

147

STAGE 1 = STARTER CARB CYCLE FOR FIRST 30 DAYS

→ START CARB CYCLE WITH YOUR NORMAL FOODS AND ADD MORE HEALTHY CHOICES

→ EXERCISE LEVEL 1: WORKOUT FOR 15-30 MINUTES DAILY

CARB CYCLE: Start by cutting all Basic Carbs in half on Mon/Tue/Thur/Fri/Sat and eat them normally on Wed/Sat-Eve/Sun. Start paying more attention to what food choices you eat and switch to more healthy choices while doing your first couple of Carb Cycles.

EXERCISE: Start walking every day for 15 minutes and do a simple 7 minute toning & stretching workout 2-4 times per week. Another option is to workout 7-10 minutes in the AM and 7-10 minutes in the PM or Evening. Optionally, for an extra fat-burn kick: 2-3 times a week, add a 7-15 Minute Walk first thing in the morning right after getting up. Drink water before and eat breakfast right after.

STAGE 2 = INTERMEDIATE CARB CYCLE FOR SECOND 30 DAYS

→ CARB CYCLE YOUR FOODS AND CHANGE TO MOSTLY HEALTHY CHOICES

→ EXERCISE LEVEL 2: WORKOUT FOR 30-60 MINUTES DAILY

CARB CYCLE: Keep your Carb Cycle by cutting basic carbs 50% on your low-carb days while switching to mostly healthy food choices, especially from Monday to Saturday.

EXERCISE: Do a cardio session - such as walking, biking, hiking, elliptical, etc - 1 time daily for 30 minutes or 2 times daily for 15 minutes. Add a 15-30 minute toning workout 3-5 times a week, ideally on Mo/Tu/Thu/Fri to further empty your carb storage on your low-carb days. Stretch out a little before, between, and after your workouts. For an extra metabolism & fat-burn kick: try to add 15 minutes of empty stomach cardio first thing in the morning 3-5 times a week. Keep this Stage for 30 days or as long as you like, then either switch to Stage 3. Advanced Carb Cycle, in order to maximize your program and chisel down even more, or go directly to Stage 4, Carb Cycle for Life, which is explained in Chapter 10 of "Franco Carlotto's Carb Cycle" Book.

STAGE 3 = ADVANCED CARB CYCLE (OPTIONAL AFTER STAGES 1 & 2)

➤ CARB CYCLE: TEMPORARILY MAXIMIZE YOUR CARB CYCLE BY
   CUTTING CARBS UP TO 75% ON LOW-CARB DAYS

➤ EXERCISE LEVEL 3: WORKOUT 60 MINUTES OR MORE DAILY

CARB CYCLE: Cut down your basic carbs from 50% to 75% on low-carb days. Never go below 50 - 75 grams/day and never skip Normal-Carb Days to refill your storage accordingly! Change to only healthy food choices, especially from Mon-Sat. Cut cheating with processed, sugary, and fatty foods, or limit to a minimum. Instead load-up with mostly healthy foods such as fruits and other natural, healthy choices on the week-ends.

EXERCISE: Ideally split up your workouts in 2-3 daily segments. For example do a 15-30 min empty stomach morning workout, another 15 min one midday, and another 15-30 one in the evening. Do cardio for at least 30-45 minutes every day, mostly at a medium intensity pace except 2-3 times a week at a higher pace. Toning or weight workouts should be done every day for 15-30 minutes or every other day for 30-60 minutes. After toning up with Stage 1 and Stage 2 - this Stage can get you in absolute Bikini Shape whenever you are ready for it by using Stage 1 and 2 firsthand. NEVER GO TO THIS STAGE IF YOU ARE A STARTER OR RE-STARTING! Remember, to lose fat and achieve top shape is a journey, not a sprint, in order to maintain it for a lifetime & keep results steady.